Hea ...
and Harmonious

BALANCING YOUR PET'S CHAKRAS

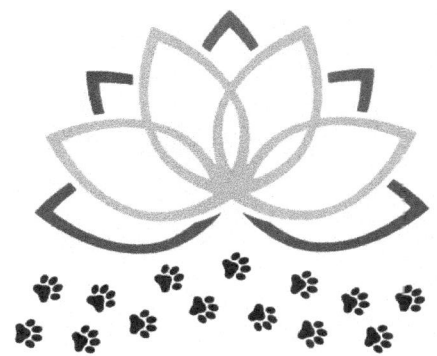

Vicki Draper

Vi Miere
Bothell, Washington

Author: Vicki Draper

Publisher: Vi Miere, Bothell, Washington

Website: HealingYourAnimal.com

Photos: by Jill Labberton, Marika Moffitt with Dirtie Dog Photography, Whole Cat and Kaboodle, pet parents, or Vicki Draper unless otherwise stated.

Lotus icon used with credit to the artist, hati.royani from vecteezy.com.

Editing and Layout: Positively Powered Publications

Cover Design: Melody Christian of Finicky Fox Designs

Healthy, Free and Harmonious: Balancing Your Pet's Chakras/ Vicki Draper. First edition.

ISBN 978-0-9976350-2-7

Five Important Things Your Vet Won't Tell You

Download this free gift from:
HealingYourAnimal.com/#freegift

You know the benefits of veterinarian care. What you may not realize is there is complimentary care that is optimal for the well-being of your pet.

Listening to this gift, *Five Important Things Your Vet Won't Tell You,* is going to open your awareness to 5 additional factors that impact your pet's health.

This free resource will help you be a more effective pet guardian and make a big difference in the quality of your pet's life.

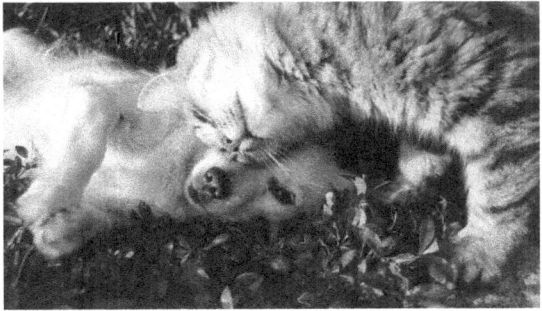

Photo from pexels.com by Snapwire

Foreword

I've been working in cat rescue for about 25 years. In that time, I have realized more about what I did not know than what I did know. It took many years for me to unlearn things and to allow myself to be retaught by the cats themselves.

My early rescue career involved the most fundamental aspect of rescue: trap, neuter, return (TNR). TNR is the most fundamental element of rescue because it addresses overpopulation at its very core. Statistics claim that over a seven-year period, two cats of reproductive age will create 420,000 offspring. That is a daunting number. I am fortunate to live in the Pacific Northwest, where we have many resources for low-cost spay/neuter options. In fact, the first free-standing feral cat clinic was established in my home city of Seattle.

During my time working with feral colonies doing both TNR and colony maintenance, I became aware of the fact that there are very few if any resources outside of low-cost clinics for feral cats. Encroachment, animal cruelty, and limited volunteer resources displace hundreds of feral cats in our area every year. In response, we opened the Feral Cat Sanctuary in 2000 and became a 501c3 in 2004.

TNR is one of two critical aspects of rescue. The other I did not learn until much later. Over the years I have worked in the pet industry and have learned so much about pet foods. I had never really thought about what I was feeding my cat. But I learned about how feeding an obligate carnivore—animals whose diet consists of at least 70 percent meat (What is a carnivore?, 2018)—a dry, overly processed diet causes not only physical problems but also behavioral problems. This, I learned, is the second fundamental aspect of rescue. A vast majority of cats are surrendered to shelters for avoidable reasons. Top among them are the behavioral problems caused by dehydration, limited resources, synthetic preservatives, and underfeeding.

When I was lucky enough to open my own cat-related business, I began teaching these concepts to anyone and everyone who came to the sanctuary looking to surrender a cat or to solve a problem. We adopt out around 300 cats per year from our little store. Most of the cats that we take in need some form of rehabilitation before they can be adopted into new homes. Rehabilitation is a three-step process. The first step is to have the cat seen by a veterinarian to rule out or factor in any physical issues. The second step is to return the cat to a species-appropriate diet—raw food and maybe some canned food. Our third step is to address the metaphysical needs of the cat.

Vicki Draper is skilled in both communication and hands-on therapy. When she works with our "broken" cats, she is able to hear what they want, and let them know that they are safe with us. Her hands-on abilities to move energy, release blocks, and read areas of pain in the cat's body give us the edge that we need to really help these cats.

Many, many times, these cats come to us completely shut down. They won't make eye contact, they won't eat, they will not use the litter box and will urinate in their own beds. They do not understand what has happened and why they have been taken from their homes and have landed in a strange place with strange sounds and smells. Many, many times Vicki has been our only hope for a breakthrough. And even though it may take her a few sessions, she has never let us down.

Her second book, *Heart to Heart,* is a big seller at our store. Her approach to connecting with your pet allows for a much deeper and better understanding of your pet's needs. It's broken down into easy to read, easy to apply segments. I love how comprehensive it is!

Vicki is an amazing source of non-traditional modalities. She covers everything that traditional veterinary work does not. From massage to reiki and acupressure, to the creation of her own crystal essences, she leaves no healing stone unturned.

Her newest book on chakras is another triumph in exploring metaphysical opportunities for health and balance. I have done work with chakras in my past, but never really thought about animals having chakras. I always associated these with ego work but never knew that they actually interface with the endocrine system! So it was fascinating to learn about the chakra system in cats and how Vicki works with them to help create balanced-based healing. I also learned so much from this book about healing my own chakra system.

I also know Vicki to be an amazing parent and pet parent. She truly comes from a place of love, peace, and joy. I'm honored to have been invited to write this foreword, if only as a way of thanking Vicki for being an integral part of our rehabilitation team and making a new life possible for so many seemingly hopeless cats. She never gives up.

—Nancy Howard, Owner of The Whole Cat and Kaboodle, Redmond, Washington

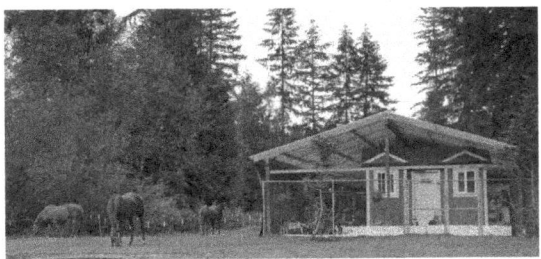

Feral Care Sanctuary , Nancy Howard, Founder

QR Code: 3D Viewing of Vicki Doing a Healing Session with Cat Opie in The Whole Cat and Kaboodle Cat Cafe

Contents

Dedication

This book is dedicated to all the human, wild, and domestic animal teachers along my way in my life.

I have been privileged to play a key role in helping thousands of people and their pets over the course of my lifetime, especially in my career.

I was born a natural healer and animal communicator. I did not have a mentor to help me cultivate my skills. It was the animals that taught me along the way, until many years later when I aligned with helping people and their pets as a career. Professional training gave me language for what I was naturally doing with the animals, along with new skills.

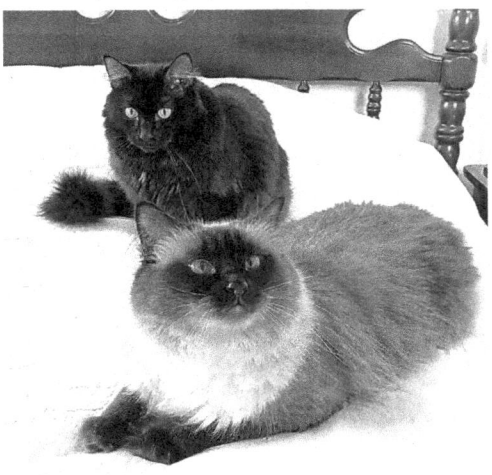

Spirit and Sapphire are Seven-Year-Old Siblings that are My Current Teachers Living with Me

Spirit is a Reiki Master who signed up to be an assistant in my healing practice. Spirit frequently joins my Zoom conversations.

Sapphire is Reiki II attuned and likes being in the background. She occasionally steps up to help with sessions or classes; however, that is not her focus or preference when being with me.

Here's a fun photo of Spirit and Sapphire "helping" as I was writing this book. I say "helping" as I had to get creative to have them on my lap and write at the same time.

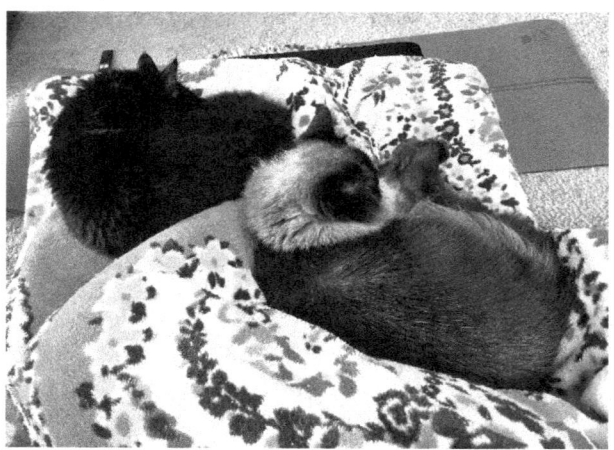

Spirit and Sapphire "Helping" Me

CHAPTER 1

What are Chakras?

THE CHAKRAS ARE AN ANCIENT ENERGY SYSTEM that originated in India. They were first mentioned in the Vedas, ancient sacred texts of spiritual knowledge that are the first texts of Hinduism, dating from 1500 to 1000 BC.

The Hindu language doesn't have an "ah" sound, so chakra is pronounced *chuh-kruh.*

Chakra (cakra in Sanskrit) means wheel.

Chakras are energy centers, vortices of light, sometimes called wheels or disks of light in your and your pet's bodies. There are seven main chakras in the body that run along the spine from the base of the spine to the crown of the head.

The chakras correspond to bundles of nerves, major organs, and areas of the energetic body that affect your and your pet's emotional and physical well-being. From the physical aspect, all chakras manage a certain part of the body, and they are connected to your and your pet's endocrine glands.

The chakras also emit color vibrations depending on the shape and intensity of the energy of each chakra. The colors and functions of the pet chakra system are similar to the human chakra system.

Lotus is a sacred symbol in Hindu philosophies. If you look closely at the chakra symbols, you will see lotus petals unfolding. The folding and unfolding of lotus petals are synonymous with the folding and unfolding of consciousness and awareness.

When the chakras are open and flowing, your and your pet's emotional and physical health are balanced. When the chakras are congested, stagnant, or blocked, that is when emotional and physical issues are present. With pets, you may see out-of-balance chakras expressed by behavioral issues as well as physical issues. Keeping your and your pet's chakras balanced, open, and flowing promotes optimum health and well-being.

Note: In the northern hemisphere, the chakras spin in a clockwise direction. In the southern hemisphere, the chakras spin in a counterclockwise direction.

Why Do We Want to Know about Chakras?

Since you made the decision to be your pet's guardian, to take the best care of them, it is important for you to realize your pet has chakras and to learn how to take care of them. By reading this book, you are on the path to doing your best and keeping your precious pet healthy.

The chakras are spinning energies in our system that keep us and our pets balanced. Chakras are continually spinning and continually working with you and your pet as you live your lives. Things that impact chakras are diet, experiences, and environment. Every experience in your daily living impacts the body and impacts the chakras, so they can easily get out of balance.

The chakras have a normal rhythm that sometimes needs help getting back into balance after a disruption. You will learn how to tell if your pet's chakras are in or out of balance and how to balance each of the chakras.

There are seven main chakras in the body along with additional chakras in your and your pet's body. I will focus on the seven main chakras with information on some of the additional chakras for your pets.

How the Chakra System Works

You and your pet have seven main chakras that go from the first chakra, the root chakra, up the body to the seventh, the crown or top of the head. The chakras are wheels of light that spin, starting from the ground (root, chakra 1) upward. What affects the first chakra impacts and feeds the rest of the chakra system. Opening and balancing the first chakra, starts the energy, spiraling up the chakra system for more opening and harmonizing with all the chakras.

No one chakra is more important than another. They all affect your and your pet's well-being.

The chakras are proportional to the size of the animal. They will be smaller for the smaller cats and dogs and larger for the larger dogs. The locations of the body, organs, and glands the chakras correspond to are the same for all size pets.

By the end of reading this book, you will be able to:

- Understand grounding.

- Balance your seven main chakras.

- Understand the seven main chakras of your pet.

- Assess the seven main chakras of your pet to determine whether they are in or out of balance.

- Understand how to use a pendulum.

- Balance each of the seven main chakras of your pet.

- Chart your progress to discover patterns with your pet's chakras.

CHAPTER 2

My Journey with the Chakras

FROM THE MOMENT I TOOK MY FIRST YOGA CLASS and heard about chakras, I wanted to learn more.

In 2000, I enrolled in a chakra class where we spent an hour per chakra over a series of seven classes on the human chakras. In each class, we learned about each chakra's location, meaning, color, physical glands, emotions, and health impacts. Then we dove deep into experiencing each of the seven main chakras in the body over the course of seven weeks. We paired up and sat face-to-face, taking turns with our partner reading the other's designated chakra that we were studying. It was interesting feeling the energy of my partner and receiving information about what she was carrying in her chakra. And when it was time to switch, to have my partner read my chakra and relate the information she received was fascinating. It was an eye-opening experience to realize how much information is stored in our bodies from our experiences. I was fascinated. I realized the importance of keeping chakras balanced and flowing healthily and harmoniously for myself and others. Later, I had the awakening that the chakras correlated to pets too.

During my Reiki training, chakras appeared again, as Reiki works with the chakras. My understanding deepened. The chakra system contains the health of the whole body.

Since my Reiki certifications Level I, II, and Master/Teacher, chakras have stayed a focus in my life and my life's work with people and their pets. I realized pets have chakras and how the quality of the basics—food, water, shelter, along with the quality of their environment, life situations, and guardian's chakras—play a role in the quality of the pet's chakras and overall health.

A benefit of Reiki and chakra balancing that my cat, Spirit, taught me is Reiki enhances grounding for people and animals.

According to physics, the definition of grounding is the process of *removing* the excess charge on an object by means of the transfer of electrons between it (in this case you and your emotions, or your pet and your pet's emotions) and another object of substantial size (in this case the Earth).

You will learn more about how to ground and the importance of grounding as you read this book.

Being a Reiki Master/Teacher, my working with the chakras is energy healing, where I am a conduit, a facilitator, allowing the all-knowing universal life-force energy to flow through me to the cat, dog, and person for the highest possible outcome of the recipient.

The stories I share are where I was a catalyst. I facilitated the healing sessions, allowing the pets' bodies' self-healing mechanisms to kick in and do the healing. This is the place where miracles and great results can take place.

I love teaching and empowering you, your pet's parent, ways to provide optimum healing care to your precious pet.

Some of the classes I teach using the chakras are Reiki Level I, II, and Master/Teacher certification classes for people and pets.

I also teach a Pet Chakra Class for balancing your pet's and your chakras whether you are new to chakras, familiar with them, or after being initiated into Reiki. In this class, we focus an hour class on each chakra for deeper learning.

This book is based on the first level of the Pet Chakra Class, which students love. They are eagerly ready for this book to be available.

Animals and nature are passions of mine. Both are a big part of my teachings. In nature are crystals and minerals that I have combined and formulated into two lines of natural healing essences called Healing You (formerly known as Vi Miere) and Healing Your Animal (HYA) Essences. In each chakra chapter you will see a Healing Your Animal Essence that balances each chakra.

I continue to deepen my knowledge and experience with the chakras to provide my best to my calling and purpose of helping people and pets live their best lives.

As part of this calling, I wrote this book to help you with your journey of discovering or deepening your knowledge and experience with the chakras for you and your precious pet(s).

CHAPTER 3

About Chakra Healing

ANIMALS ARE PRECIOUS, RESPECTED BEINGS TO ME. I like honoring each animal as their special unique being. Animals are a very important part of my household and are treated accordingly.

I want to share why it is important for me to use the terms "pet guardian" or "pet parent" rather than "pet owner."

We adopt our pet and have them live with us, so we are a "parent," or the guardian of the pet. We provide a good life for our pet(s). And we want them to be happy, healthy, and harmonious, living their best lives.

You will hear me use the terms "pet guardian" or "pet parent" throughout this book as a sign of respect for our pet(s).

Humans and animals are electromagnetic beings, which means we all have the conscious choice and healing capacity to do chakra balancing with our pet.

Anyone reading this book can utilize the techniques taught here and do chakra balancing.

For those of you who haven't heard about chakras or don't know much about the chakras, this book is a great place to start. Welcome to this new exploration that can healthily change your and your pet's life.

For those of you who say to yourself, "I already know all about the chakras," I ask that you be open, as there is always more to learn.

Since you are here, I suspect that is the case with you. You are open, ready to learn or review while gaining new insights.

You may know about the chakras for humans. Do you know about chakras and how they relate to your pets? Chakras relating to your pets is a different insight that I am delighted to be sharing with you.

There is a lot of information available on human chakras that you can easily find.

This book is focused primarily on your pet's chakras, going deeply with each of the seven main chakras on your pet. You are included in a chapter dedicated to you and your chakras.

You have heard me mention Reiki. The next step working with the chakras is Reiki.

Why Reiki?

Here's why it is important to share some information with you.

Everyone who has taken Reiki is working with the chakras.

Reiki is composed of two Japanese words: "rei" meaning universal and "ki" meaning life force energy. It is a form of energy healing.

Reiki is important if you are interested in becoming a healer for people and/or animals and will enhance the chakra experience.

There are three different certification levels to Reiki, as follows:

Reiki Level 1: The ability to heal oneself.

Reiki Level 2: The ability to heal oneself and others.

Reiki Level 3: The ability to heal oneself and others and teach the technique to students.

Each level gives you deeper, stronger access to the Reiki healing.

Reiki Level 1 you learn the Reiki hand positions.

Reiki Level 2 you learn the Reiki symbos and how to use them. This opens your ability to do distance healing when you are away from your pet or loved ones.

Reiki Level 1 and Level 2 are a good combination for most people's personal use.

Reiki Master is recommended for people wanting to incorporate Reiki healing into their professional practice.

The Reiki study conducted at Harvard University by members of the Center for Reiki Research (Dr. Natalie Dyer, Dr. Ann Baldwin, and William Rand) in 2015 and 2016 has now been published in the *Journal of Alternative and Complementary Medicine.* This is the largest prospective Reiki study to date and hopefully will lead to much more research.

The Harvard study with 1,411 Reiki practitioners concluded that a single session of Reiki improves multiple variables related to physical and psychological health.

For more information on Reiki, visit:

HealingYourAnimal.com/Reiki.php.

Wherever you are on your journey with the chakras, I hope you and your pet(s) enjoy your experience with this book.

Some Things to Keep in Mind

Healing does not always mean miraculous, instantaneous rebounding from an illness. Healing is a process. Sometimes it requires multiple chakra balancing sessions. Sometimes one chakra balancing session can make a big impact, and other times the chakra balancing sessions are about providing comfort, support, and natural pain relief as you or your pet navigate what is happening.

Sometimes with healing, it may appear that things are getting worse and then shifts to getting better. The chakra balancing brings forward what is already in the body for it to release and heal. We are going into the root of issues to heal them.

An example is an infected wound on your body. The infection needs to come out. (In this scenario, hopefully you are seeing your doctor for medical support as well.) As you work with the body, the infection gets stirred up because it is being asked to shift and release out of the body. The pain, infection, and inflammation must find their way out of the body, so it may feel worse and more intense initially. As it is clearing your body, you start to feel better. When it does leave, you feel better than when you started.

This happens when we have an infection and take an antibiotic.

When antibiotics kill bacteria, they release poisonous toxins, which often makes you feel worse before you start to feel better.

This is called the Herxheimer response. According to Holtorf Medical Group, the Herxheimer response is a natural bodily process triggered by a greater prevalence of endotoxins. These substances are released when harmful microorganisms and bacteria are destroyed or die off. As damaging bacteria are destroyed, they release previously contained endotoxins into the bloodstream. This allows the toxins to be transported to the appropriate system and subsequently expelled from the body. However, rapid destruction of bacteria can cause an influx of endotoxins resulting in greater toxicity. When this occurs, the immune system responds by triggering an acute immune response resulting in inflammation that may be experienced throughout the body. This can cause worsening of current symptoms and the development of new symptoms.

The Herxheimer reaction is frequently seen during antibiotic treatments because antibiotics destroy numerous microorganisms and bacteria. Although the Herxheimer reaction is typically non-lethal, it does frequently cause temporary pain, discomfort, and worsening of symptoms. Symptom severity is often indicative of the level of inflammation triggered by the immune system.

This is a physical example, but the same can apply to behavioral and emotional situations too.

When your two- and four-legged family is carrying so much stress, and the healing starts happening, it may escalate unwanted behaviors, because the status quo is changing, like a hornet's nest being stirred up. This means progress even though it looks and feels more chaotic at the time of healing.

Think of your family as each member being a piece of a hanging mobile. When you touch one piece of the mobile, all the pieces are affected and move until they find a new balance.

We are working at the core; things will get stirred up and things will balance out in a much better place than when the healing started.

Here is an example of working with behavioral issues. I was working recently with a Krissy, the guardian of five cats named Mama, Mini Me, Felix, Oscar, and Squints, and one dog named Zorro. Cats Mama, Mini Me, and Felix started not getting along; a separate issue is the dog must be separated from the cats. Krissy desires harmony in her home and with all four-legged members. This is clearly a case that involved multiple sessions to get to the root and have all family members feeling harmonious.

The first session focused on Felix, the cat who was getting bullied and beat up on by Mama and sometimes Mini Me. The idea was that chakra balancing would help Felix so that when he feels more balanced and confident, he won't be a target. During this first session, Mini Me was very calm and settled at the beginning, but he was running around unsettled the whole time the healing energy was present. This was totally out of character for Mini Me. He was feeling the energy shift with their family dynamic (in other words, the mobile pieces were moving, and he was being affected).

The next session, the plan was to work with Mama, who was very upset and the main instigator of picking on Felix. Between sessions, because of a heat wave, the cats needed to be moved inside to air-conditioning from their cozy, unairconditioned "catio."

Felix was very calm and solid from the balancing he had received the week before. He handled this move with ease. Oscar had become very ungrounded and out of sorts with the change. I balanced his root chakra and helped him settle, and I then started working with Mama as planned. I discovered that Mama was harboring a lot of stress and grumpiness. She had been on her own having to struggle to survive before coming into her new forever home with Krissy. Mama's angst with Felix was coming from a trigger in Mama from this experience. As Mama was balancing, her stressed energy was dissipating. Mama's demeanor was softening and calming. Balancing Mama's root chakra helped settle her attitude with Felix.

You will learn more about the root chakra as you read further in the book, especially Chapter 5, "Root Chakra."

I am sharing this portion of a complex situation as an example of healing, starting with a core issue and working our way out to total harmony with life events happening along the way.

Healing is a process, not an instant solution. By being patient and going through the process where things may get stirred up before getting better, know that there is a more harmonious life for this family on the other side of this healing process.

After a series of healing sessions with Krissy and her cats, Mama, Mini Me, and Felix, the cats can be in the same room together. The fighting mellowed. Mama cat now sits calmly in Krissy's lap (she had not done that before the healing sessions). There is more harmony between the cats in the household and a deeper bonding with Mama and Krissy.

Energy is not linear, which means it is not an exact science. Energy works with vibrations, feelings, pictures, and flow.

Working with the chakras is working with the energies in your and your pet's bodies. There are some differences in correlations with organs and chakras depending on what chakra system is being referenced.

I am sharing from the system that correlates with my chakra and acupressure training. Acupressure is from traditional Chinese medicine (TCM), which has been around for centuries. (Other systems may describe chakras differently.)

I invite you to find what information aligns with you, keep it, and leave the rest. Explore what is true for you.

Note: An important thing to keep in mind is healing and balancing chakras don't replace the need for veterinarian care.

For example, you will discover in Chapter 6 that the second chakra is associated with the urinary tract. If your cat has crystals in their urinary tract, the crystals may cause a blockage; your cat may need surgery. Your pet needs veterinary care to remove the blockage. In this case, supporting the second chakra helps with pain relief, preparing your pet for the surgery, and supporting your pet with recovery after the surgery. Using veterinarian care and chakra healing together provides the best quality of care for your pet.

The one thing that is certain is balancing your chakras and your pet's balances both bodies and is a healthy thing to do regularly for wellness and promoting optimal health for you and your pet.

That is my intention for writing this book: sharing support for optimal health for you and your pet for your lives together.

I am privileged to be part of the rehabilitation support team for a local cat store, Whole Cat and Kaboodle, Redmond,

Washington, and Feral Care Sanctuary, Bothell, Washington. Nancy Howard is the owner and founder of both facilities.

They take in cats that have been in some rough situations, guardians going to euthanize them instead of getting help, guardians passing away with cats having rowhere to go, and more.

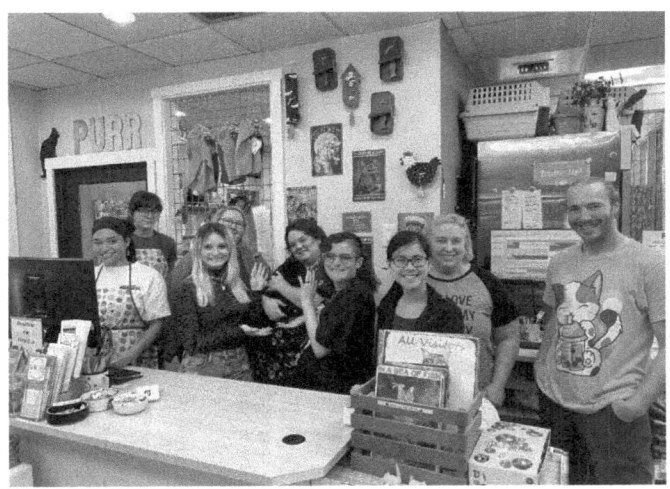

Whole Cat and Kaboodle Team

I know when Nancy calls me in there is a cat or cats in dire straits, because Nancy and her team are very skilled and adept in helping distressed cats rehabilitate. Sometimes, the cats need the healing, chakra balancing, and communication I offer to be the catalyst that shifts them into recovery.

After recovery, the cats are adopted into their new forever homes.

I am honored to be a part of the rehabilitation team and to feature some of these stories in this book as teaching examples.

QR Code: 3D Viewing of Vicki Doing a Healing Session with Cat Opie in The Whole Cat and Kaboodle Cat Cafe

Now that you have learned about the chakras for you and your pets, let's look at another aspect of chakras, how your chakras affect your pet's chakras.

CHAPTER 4

Relationship between Pet's and Guardian's Chakras

OUR PETS LIVE WITH US IN OUR ENVIRONMENT. We have domesticated them and brought them into the human home. It's important to realize what happens in this scenario with the chakras for both the pet and the guardian.

How Pet Guardian's Chakras Affect Their Pet's Chakras

Our pets take on our issues. They do it because they are constantly in our environment, and they care about us. This is why it is good to do daily clearing techniques and have professional maintenance support on a regular basis.

What you may not realize is that the quality of your chakras as your pet's guardian affects the quality of your pet's health. Your chakras are energy centers emanating out into your environment, where your pet lives with you. Your pet is constantly feeling this as energy information and taking it into their chakras.

When your pet is anxious, unsettled, and what you call "misbehaving," it may be because you, their guardian, and/or their environment are chaotic. Animals react to the energy around them. They need an outlet to process the unsettled energy. The good news is that this book will help you with this. I encourage you to pay close attention to the grounding sections for you and your pet.

Dog Calms When Guardian Grounds

Peggy came to see me because of her dog Cato's aggression issues toward her. She was afraid of being around Cato, not knowing when his aggression issues would arise and she would get bitten.

I could see Cato was very anxious, and Peggy was as well. So, the first thing I did was help Peggy ground herself.

As I was walking Peggy through this grounding process, Cato's demeanor shifted from standing and on edge to lying down, calm, and relaxed. Peggy was stunned to discover the connection between her energy and Cato's response in his behavior. See Chapter 13 for how to do a grounding exercise.

Importance of Conscious Petting and Connecting with Your Pet

One impact on your pet's chakras that is coming from you is when you are not conscious about how your energy affects them. For example, you have your day, you come home, you bend down or pick up your pet, loving on them, connecting, petting, and hugging your pet. The whole time, you may be unconsciously releasing all the heavy energy from your day. They're just happily taking it all from you because they love you and want to help you. You feel better, but now your pet has to process this excess energy. Sometimes they can release it easily. When they cannot, that starts a build-up of heavy energy in their system that begins to take a toll on your pet's behavior and physical body.

When you manage your energy, you keep your pet healthier and happier.

In physics, you are the larger object, the larger energy field, so it is stronger and has more of an impact on the environment (including your pet) than your pet's impact on the environment with his/her energy field. (The exception may be if you are a very small person and you have a large breed, your energy may be more even with your pet. Still, your pet is generally more open and therefore more susceptible to taking on your energy than vice versa.)

Your pet likes to help you. It is important to help your pet process and clear what is yours because they are taking it on to help you. Check out Chapter 13: "Preparing You" to learn how to do chakra balancing for yourself to help keep your energies clean and balanced.

Dog Helping Guardian after Surgery

Sheri has been a client for 12 years and Farrah is her fourth whippet we have worked together with.

Sheri knows the value of having regular healing sessions to navigate life's journey with Farrah. She pays for monthly sessions a year in advance, so we keep Farrah's energy maintained on a monthly basis for her best health.

Quote from Sheri: "I am someone who wants to know how to inhabit a fuller relationship with my dog and to have more access to what she thinks and feels and needs so that I can do my part to make sure she has everything she needs."

Remember what I shared earlier: Our pets take on our issues. They do it because they are in our environment, and they care about us.

During one session, Sheri had surgery on her left upper arm since our previous month's session.

What I discovered was Farrah had been helping Sheri recover from her surgery and had literally taken on Sheri's pain.

During Farrah's healing session, Farrah released the pain energy in her upper front left leg.

The healing session provided the space for Farrah's healing to take place. Sheri's hurt energy was released from Farrah, and Farrah's energy flow was full and vibrant again.

And to help Farrah know her mom was being taken care of, Sheri received healing support from me too along with Farrah in the healing session. This made Farrah very happy.

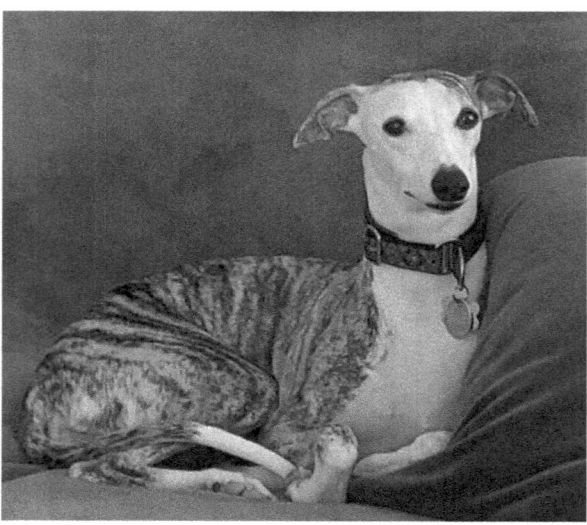

Farrah

Puppies Helping with Right Hip Pain

My client, Kim, had two eleven-month-old puppies, Biscuit and Brulee, that were receiving wellness sessions. In one session, I noticed Biscuit had right hip energy that needed clearing. I thought maybe he tweaked it playing until I worked with Brulee. When I was working with Brulee, she also had right hip issues showing up to clear. Now, this was unusual for both puppies to have the same issue at the same time. That is when I looked to Kim and asked, "Are you having right hip pain?" She said, "Oh yes, it has been acting up and is really bothering me." Biscuit and Brulee were helping Kim with her pain, and it was getting stuck in their bodies.

It is common for our pets to take on our "stuff." It is important for us to stay as healthy as possible and to do regular wellness clearing, centering, and protection as taught in my first book, *Bridging True Love Connection & Healing Between You and Your Animals*, along with chakra balancing. Because we are close to our pets, it is important to stay as neutral as possible, with no attachment, when working with our pets for the best results. Let go of any agenda. Let go of what you know so you are open to the experience and the information you receive.

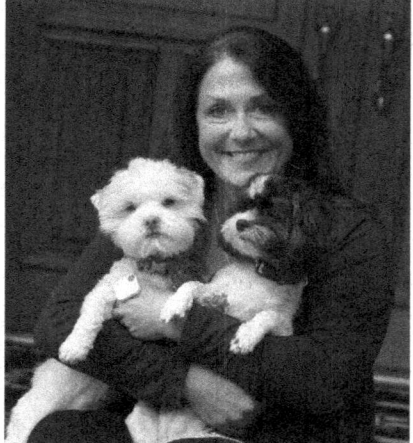

Kim, Biscuit, and Brulee

Digestion Issues in Pet from Guardian

Rocky, a black Labradoodle, is a regular client. This means I know his energy very well.

He was a picky eater and was having digestive issues a few sessions in a row. He would get better after his session and then have digestive issues again.

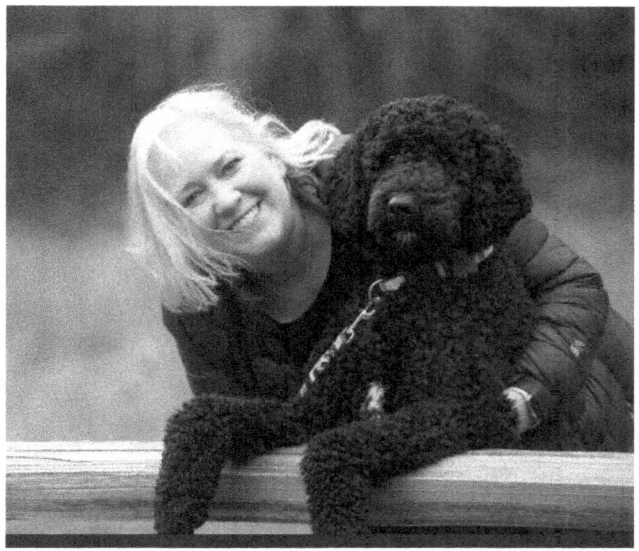

Heidi and Rocky

It was then that I asked Heidi, his guardian, "How is your digestion?" Her response was, "Ohhhh." Bingo! She realized she was having digestion issues. This was a case where we had to focus on supporting Heidi, the guardian's digestive issues, to help heal Rocky's digestive issues.

How a Pet's Chakras May Affect a Guardian's Chakras

A situation where your chakras are affected by your pet is if you are very energy sensitive and take on your pet's energy because of your deep connection.

Another instance is when your pet is not feeling well and you are worried sick, you feel sick or your heart aches as you see your pet not feeling well. Or you feel deep guilt that your pet doesn't feel well. This may disrupt your eating, your sleeping habits, and your chakras.

Dog's Upset Stomach Issue Caused Guardian Stomach Issue

Lenny was worried about her dog, Stan. He was sluggish, sleeping a lot, and had a poor appetite. She had taken Stan to multiple veterinarians trying to get a diagnosis with no luck. But something was clearly going on with him.

Lenny and Stan have a very close relationship. When Stan is not feeling well, Lenny physically does not feel well. Her emotions and worry over Stan made her stomach upset, and she was having trouble with eating and sleeping.

I discovered Stan had a lot of energetic upset in his third chakra, the digestive area. There was some of Lenny's upset energy in Stan's third chakra as well that he was able to release. Even with Stan not feeling well, he was helping Lenny. That's what our pets do for us.

They were energetically feeding off each other. When Stan wasn't feeling well and not eating, Lenny's stomach got upset, and she couldn't eat.

Stan was taking on Lenny's third chakra digestive issues because he didn't like seeing her in emotional and physical pain. They were in a loop of energy, supporting each other while contributing to an imbalance for both of their third chakras.

After Stan's session, Lenny reported that was he perked up, had more energy, and was eating. Lenny's stomach and digestive issues cleared up too.

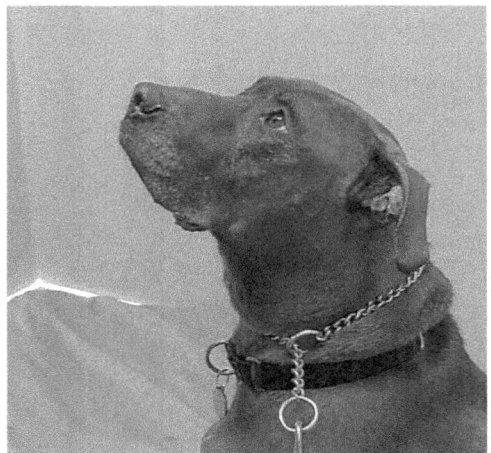

Stan

Your Pet Is a Great Barometer/Mirror for You

One student in my Pet Chakra Class, Tatyana, noticed how the more she's practicing grounding, the less startled her canine companion, Cooper, is to noises in his environment. Previously, he would hear something, get up, and leave her side. Now he is sticking around her more.

Heidi and Rocky Grounding Story

Heidi was frustrated when going on walks with Rocky, a 79-pound Labradoodle. She was not able to contain Rocky's attention when he would see a squirrel or something that piqued his interest. I suggested to Heidi to try grounding before taking Rocky out for his walks. When she did, she immediately noticed Rocky was looking at her, waiting for direction instead of wanting to shoot out straight ahead. It wasn't until she was grounded that Rocky considered Heidi the leader. It was a simple, subtle shift that made a big difference.

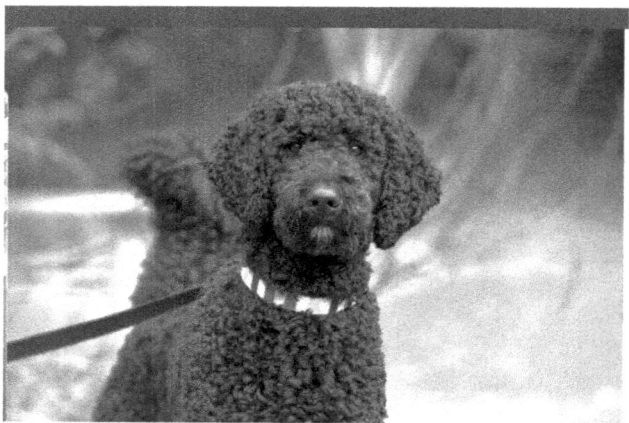

Rocky

Now that you understand why it's important to care about your and your pet's chakras, let's dive into learning more about each specific chakra.

CHAPTER 5

CHAPTER 5

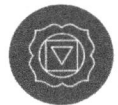

Root Chakra

THE FIRST CHAKRA IS CALLED ROOT CHAKRA, or base chakra.

This chakra is very important for you and your animal(s) because it is the foundation of all the other chakras. It represents survival and safety. Being domesticated and living with you in your home, your pets depend on you for their survival and safety, including healthy food, comfortable shelter, and a loving environment.

Color: Red

Sound: Lam (pronounced Lahm)

Musical note: C

Healing Your Animal Essence: Chakra 1, ground

Emotions: Balanced, secure, grief, depression

Organs/glands: Large intestine (colon), gall bladder, coccygeal sacral plexus, adrenals

Parts of the body: Nerves, lymph, blood, hips, lower limbs, fur/hair, bones and skeletal system, prostate, perineum, rectum, gonads

Location: The base of the spine, low back, base of tail

In balance: Your pet will feel calm, comfortable, secure, and grounded in his/her surroundings. Your pet will have a general trust of people and confidence in how they carry themself and will handle changes with ease. Your pet has a strong immune system.

Out of balance: Your pet may have trouble staying still. They are pacing, skittish, and startle easily. Your pet appears nervous and fearful and may even hide. They may not like change. Dogs may have their tails tucked up underneath them.

Also, an indication of being out of balance and not feeling safe is your pet may be resource guarding— being very protective of their food, toys, and you, their guardian.

More signs that your pet's root chakra is out of balance are aggression, lack of the will to live, not eating, inappropriate urination and/or pooping, constipation, low immunity, cancer, anemia, hip issues, and arthritis.

There is more emphasis on the root chakra for you and your pet than the other chakras because it is the foundation of the seven main chakras. It is important to understand that if your root chakra is out of balance, the other chakras will be affected. It is also important to understand how the root chakra becomes out of balance as this can be the root of a lot of issues.

How Your Root Chakra Becomes Out of Balance

The root chakra is all about sense of safety and survival. If you are not feeling safe and secure, your root chakra is going to be out of balance. If you do not feel stable in your finances, food, and shelter, your root chakra is out of balance. Your pet's root chakra will also be out of balance. They look to you for this safety and security.

For animals, it's food, shelter, and their environment. If they don't feel safe in their environment, their root chakra will have balance issues.

How Your Pet's Root Chakra Becomes Out of Balance

- Their person is not grounded.

- Their person is not feeling safe.

- Their person is feeling upset.

- Animal is in foster care or shelter.

- Animal is being adopted (changing their living situation).

- You're traveling with your animal.

- You're traveling away from your animal.

- Your pet is going to the veterinarian.

- Your pet is going to the groomer.

- Your pet is going on outings with you.

- There is construction inside the house.

- There is construction outside the house.

- You're moving home locations.

- You're having company over.

- Your child is leaving for college.

- There is a marriage in the family.

- A new baby/child/person is coming into family.

- There is a divorce.

- Days around a full moon and some eclipses.

Ungrounded to Grounded Pets

Going to the Groomer

Jane, one of the Pet Chakra Class students, has a Pomeranian dog named Scout. Scout had a problem getting car sick when riding in the car even for very short rides. When Jane learned about the root chakra, she started holding his root chakra on Scout's car rides to the veterinarian and groomer while her daughter drove. She reported noticing that it made a difference. Scout was much calmer and he didn't get sick.

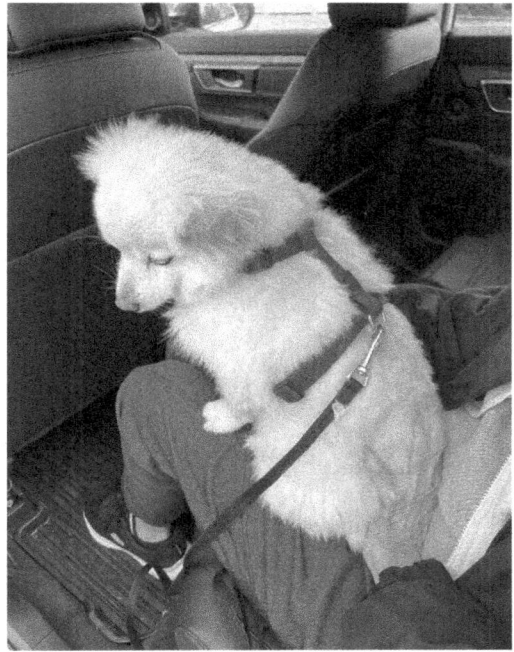

Jane Holding Scout's Root Chakra in Car

It is important to keep you and your pet safe, so do not drive while you do this technique. Use this technique only when you are a passenger and someone else is driving. This is how Jane was able to help Scout.

Going on an Outing

Karla, one of the Pet Chakra Class students, has a Shih Tzu, Havanese, Maltese mixed-breed dog named Nicky. Nicky was nervous and afraid. He was not comfortable with other people coming up to him to pet him.

Now, Karla pushes Nicky in a cart through stores while she holds his root chakra. This settles Nicky, and Karla can discourage people from approaching to keep Nicky feeling safe and secure.

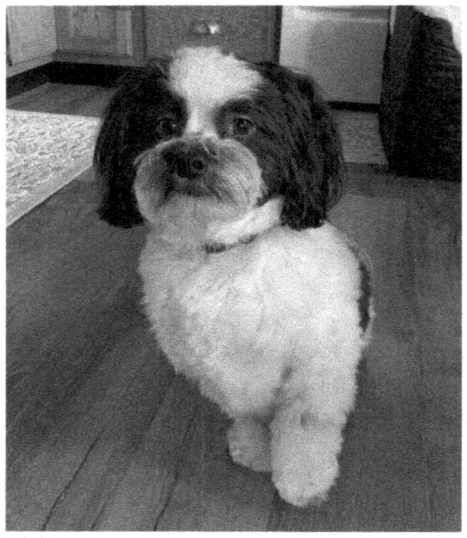

Nicky

Having Animal Company Over

Heidi is a pet guardian of a dog, Rocky, and a cat, Aslan. Heidi is a nice person with a generous soul; she's a big animal lover. She volunteered to take care of her neighbor's two dogs for a week in her home while their guardians traveled.

Heidi is a regular client who takes good care of her animals by providing monthly healing sessions with me for Rocky and Aslan to live their best lives. The benefit with this plan is that I get to know animals and their guardians very well. I know when something is out of balance that is not from normal living.

During the session after the neighbor's dogs, Ronan and Ivy, stayed with Heidi, Rocky, and Aslan n their home, Aslan's root chakra was spinning wildly out of control. This was not typical for him. He is a mild-mannered cat.

Ronan is an ungrounded dog. He is super sweet, yet he is very boisterous, like a bull in the china shop. He is all over the place, not paying attention to what is in his path, including Aslan, as he runs around enthusiastically. Living with Ronan for a week had Aslan off-balance and desiring some calm and stable energy in his environment.

Rocky usually goes first for his healing session. This session, Aslan made a beeline for the computer zoom screen, wanting his session ASAP, demanding he go first.

Aslan was out of sorts, feeling displaced with the extra dogs in his home. Aslan had been very grumpy, biting Heidi a lot and batting her with his paws.

The extra dogs in his house went on for a week. No wonder his root chakra was out of whack. He wasn't feeling safe and secure in his own home because there had been a big disruption to his routine.

Aslan loves his chakra balancing sessions. He responded well, and his root chakra calmed and got back into balance.

These stories illustrate how your environment and what goes on in your home affects your pet.

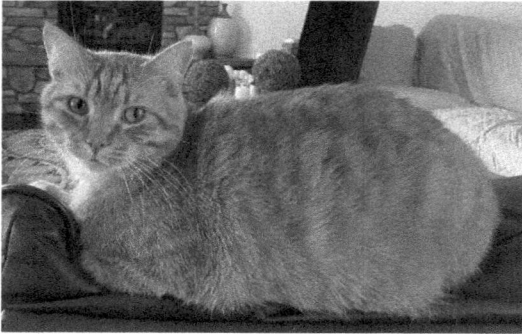

Aslan

Travel and Moving

Jenae came to see me as a private client to support her around making a permanent move from Seattle to Peru with her four pets: two Vizsla dogs, Willow and Fern, and two Bengal cats, Pax and Hunter. Their trip included a month-long stay at a beach in Peru before moving to the jungle, which would be their new, permanent home.

She wanted to make the move as easy as possible on them. She also wanted them to reinforce that they are loved and safe as they move to their new home.

- Jenae had concerns for each of them, as they all have different personalities.

- She knew their new place was going to have new experiences for all of them.

- With Willow, Jenae was concerned about her reaction meeting new dogs. Willow had previously been attacked by a dog and had since been more reactive to other dogs. And there would be dogs where they were moving.

- With Fern, she was concerned about her bladder and being able to not have an accident for the long trip.

- Jenae wasn't too concerned about Pax. She wanted him as well as the others to be as comfortable as possible.

- With Hunter, she wanted to make sure he knew he was included. She had some concern he might not navigate the trip well because he is very skittish by nature, and he might be happier staying behind. She wanted to know what Hunter's wishes were.

First, I got all four pets balanced, calm, and settled, especially making sure all their root chakras were strongly balanced. This was going to set them up for an easier travel time. They all received clear communication of what was happening step-by-step along the whole journey of their move. I had to communicate that the trip was bigger than just a few plane rides to their new home. There was the temporary month stay at the beach, ther they would fly again, have a hotel stay, and then a long bus ride to their new home.

Willow responded well to the chakra balancing, and she released the trauma from her recent dog attack.

Fern was shown the clear potty options on the flight layovers and that she would have options to pee and poop without having an accident in her kennel.

Pax received energy boosting to make sure he was ready for the long trip.

When communicating with Hunter, he made clear that he wanted to make the trip. To help Hunter with extra grounding, Jenae put a red sarong around his carrier through the airport and during car rides to protect him from the energies of the airport and travel (a good root chakra tip for you).

Hunter and Pax had to separate from Jenae and travel in cargo during one of the legs of travel. Hunter was very specific about a sacred geometrical shape and color he wanted surrounding him to protect him as well as the red sarong.

Hunter is now very happily living in the jungles of Peru with Willow, Fern, and Pax.

Willow was able to meet other dogs at their new places with ease.

Fern was able to make the trip with no peeing accidents.

And Pax made the trip easily.

The report back from Jenae was it was evident that Willow, Fern, Pax, and Hunter all were as comfortable as possible on the many legs of the trip. The preparation sessions had made a big difference. They knew they were loved, safe, and protected and going to their new home.

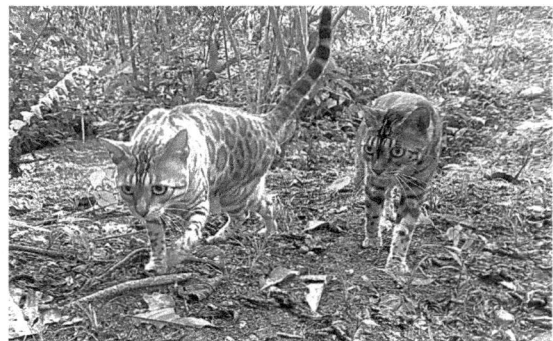

Pax and Hunter enjoying the Jungle in Peru

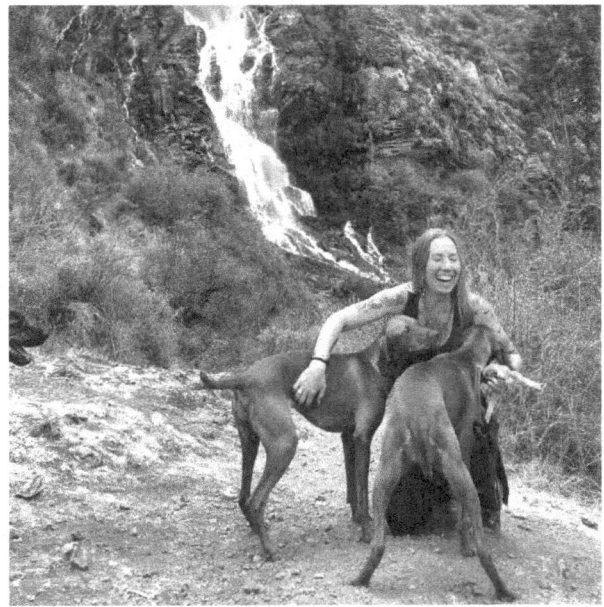

Jenae, Willow, and Fern Enjoying the Mountains of Peru

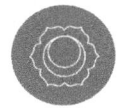

CHAPTER 6

Sacral Chakra

THE SECOND CHAKRA IS CALLED SACRAL CHAKRA, also known as the hara chakra.

This chakra is important as it is the reproductive center, which includes pleasure, sensuality, and sexuality. It is also where emotions and feelings arise. It is the center of creativity, passions, relationships, and self-worth.

Color: Orange

Sound: Vam (pronounced Vahm)

Musical note: D

Healing Your Animal Essence: Chakra 2, passion

Emotions: Playful, fear, anxiety

Organs/glands: Kidneys, bladder, prostatic plexus, spleen, reproductive organs, ovaries, adrenal gland, intestines

Parts of the body: Sacrum, lumbosacral plexus

Location:

- Back: midline over the hips on low back
- Front: just below the belly button, between the waist and pelvis

Note: Yes, your pet has a belly button, although it may be hard to find. The belly button on your pet looks like a small scar. It is flat and located in the center of the abdomen. Animal's belly buttons do not appear as innies and outies like humans'.

In balance: An animal is warm, loving, and affectionate. Note: this may look different for different cats and dogs because some may be loving and affectionate in their way that isn't as exuberant as golden retrievers who tend to be open, happy, affectionate, and loving.

Your pet may demonstrate curiosity and a desire to explore and play.

Out of balance: Pets not wanting to be petted, not wanting to connect, not interested in playing, or having separation anxiety. Animals may also be clingy, or needy, acting like Velcro, not wanting to leave your side. Spay/neuter issues, infertility, and impotence also illustrate an out-of-balance sacral chakra. Food obsession, jealousy, bladder or urinary tract infection, crystals, kidney issues, and low back pain are more signs that your pet's second chakra is out of balance.

How Your Sacral Chakra Becomes Out of Balance

The sacral chakra is all about emotions, self-worth, creativity, and sexuality. If you are not feeling sexy, sassy, and creative, your sacral chakra is going to be out of balance. If you are ridden with self-criticism and guilt, your sacral chakra is out of balance. If you have had a negative sexual experience or abuse, or emotionally charged events, your second chakra is affected.

For animals, if they are like Velcro with you, attached all the time, don't like leaving your side, their sacral charka is out of balance.

How Your Pet's Sacral Chakra Becomes Out of Balance

- Their person is feeling lots of guilt and shame.

- Their person's emotions are out of balance.

- They have had recent spay or neuter surgery.

- They have bladder/UTI, kidney issues, or crystals in the urine.

- They do not have a balanced diet that addresses all your pet's dietary needs.

- Their hormones are out of balance.

- Breeders who are trying to control the breeding process can upset the pets.

Breeding

Hattie, a Bouvier dog, was a little older, and I discovered by communicating with her that she really wanted to have puppies. So Lynn, Hattie's guardian, was going to artificially inseminate her. Lynn and I were working with the second chakra to help give Hattie a better chance of her body easily accepting being inseminated for pregnancy.

Because of the COVID-19 pandemic happening, Hattie had to wait until she was almost seven years old to be bred. Then it was near Thanksgiving, and Hattie was not able to get inseminated at the optimal time to have success with pregnancy. She really wanted to be a mom and have puppies and went into a false pregnancy.

According to Fetch by WebMD, false pregnancy is a common condition in unneutered female dogs. It's also known as pseudopregnancy, pseudocyesis, or a phantom pregnancy in dogs.

Around 80% of unspayed female dogs—those who still have their ovaries and uterus—will show some signs of a false pregnancy at least once in their lives. Around 67% will have recurring symptoms.

False pregnancy was not typical for Hattie. The veterinarian thought maybe Hattie was pregnant with one puppy early on that got reabsorbed.

Hattie ended up with a lump on her breast that may have been part of the reason not getting or staying pregnant. The lump was precancerous and was surgically removed.

Being a Bouvier breed and knowing Hattie's history, Lynn would normally have had Hattie spayed by the time she was seven years old to prevent breast cancer. Hattie having a false pregnancy may have been her body knowing what was best for her.

Nature knows best.

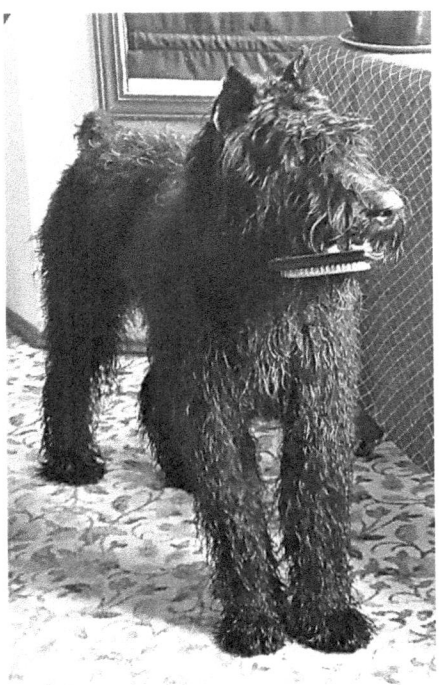

Hattie

For males, balancing the second chakra to prepare him to mate with a female can be beneficial.

Peeing Outside the Litter Box

My cat client Jax was peeing outside the litter box. When balancing his chakras, he gave me a painful response in his second chakra. I mentioned this to his guardian and recommended a veterinarian visit to get him checked out.

Unfortunately, it's difficult to detect that your cat is in pain. Cats are wired to hide any signs of pain and discomfort, a trait that they have inherited from their wild ancestors. In the wild, displaying pain shows vulnerability, which can make them prime targets of predators.

Jax's guardian asked me, "What do I say to the veterinarian?" I shared that Jax's pain was bladder related and suggested that she request a urine test. It turns out that Jax had crystals in his urine.

Crystals in the urine are medically referred to as "crystalluria." The formation of crystals in urine occurs when there is supersaturation or a high concentration of crystal-forming minerals that naturally occur in urine. These minerals can clump together and form crystals.

When crystals are present in the urine, your vet needs to establish whether crystalluria is medically significant so a treatment regimen can be formulated if necessary.

This a good example of when knowing what each chakra represents helps getting veterinarian care for your pet.

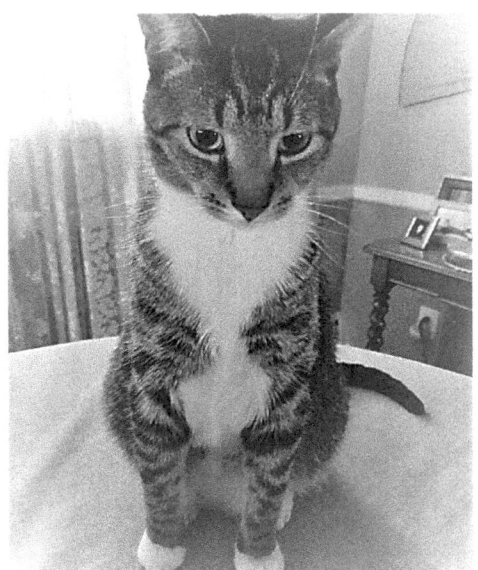

Jax

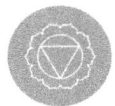

CHAPTER 7

Solar Plexus Chakra

THE THIRD CHAKRA IS CALLED THE SOLAR PLEXUS CHAKRA.

This chakra is important because it is the center of personal power, the center of will the core. It is how animals carry themselves into the world. It is the center of desires. It plays an important role in your pet's immune system.

Color: Yellow

Sound: Ram (pronounced Rahm)

Musical note: E

Healing Your Animal Essence: Chakra 3, desires

Emotions: Courage, anger

Organs/glands: Liver, gallbladder, spleen, pancreas, stomach, solar plexus

Parts of the body: Digestion system, assimilation, adrenals, diaphragm, skin (integumentary), muscles, eyesight, nervous system

Location:

- Back: mid-back

- Front: between the base of ribcage and above the navel

In balance: Your pet is full of confidence, strutting their stuff, and displaying healthy digestion and a healthy immune system.

Out of balance: Your pet is submissive, fearful, timid, and skittish. Or the opposite—your pet is being a bully, being bossy or aggressive. Your pet may have digestion issues, diabetes, pancreatitis, liver issues, immune disorders, jaundice, gall stones, hypoglycemia, hepatitis, ulcers, or skin issues.

The third chakra is a powerful chakra. It is the center of the digestive center. Just like humans', the majority of cat's and dog's immune system resides in the digestion system.

When you change your pet's food, supporting their third chakra can help make the change more easily. Changing your pet's food can cause a detoxification process while your pet's digestive tract and body are acclimating to the new food. To discover how to change foods to support them with easy transition, see my second book, *Heart to Heart: How you can heal your animal through all stages of life,* Chapter 1: "Preparing for Life with a New Pet."

Signs your pet's third chakra and digestion may be out of balance:

- Vomiting
- Diarrhea
- Constipation
- Gas
- Bloating
- Mucous poops

How Your Solar Plexus Chakra Becomes Out of Balance

The solar plexus chakra is all about your personal power, self-esteem, healthy digestion, and immunity. If you are not feeling strength in your core self, confidence, warmth, and self-control, your solar plexus chakra is going to be out of balance.

How Your Pet's Solar Plexus Chakra Becomes Out of Balance

- Their person has a lack of confidence or low self-esteem.
- They have eaten a food that is not good for them.

- They are exposed to places where they don't feel comfortable.

- They feel stress due to their person expecting too much of them.

- They have been with other animals they don't feel compatible being around.

- They lack a purpose; your pet likes helping you.

- Types of purposes: to make you laugh, to protect the house when you're away, to protect their "little brother" or "little sister," or to provide balance, etc.

- Not being stimulated enough through play or activities.

For example, a very active, high-drive dog such as a border collie that is always being told to sit still and not given an outlet for matching the dog's needs.

Dog Eats Poisonous Mushroom

Rosie, a miniature Labradoodle, had eaten a poisonous mushroom on one of her walks. Luckily, I have a friend who is a professional chef and could help identify the mushroom that Rosie ate. This helped when she got emergency veterinarian support. After that, I gave Rosie chakra balancing support to help her start eating again.

Since this incident, her digestive tract has been very sensitive. Keeping her third chakra balanced is important.

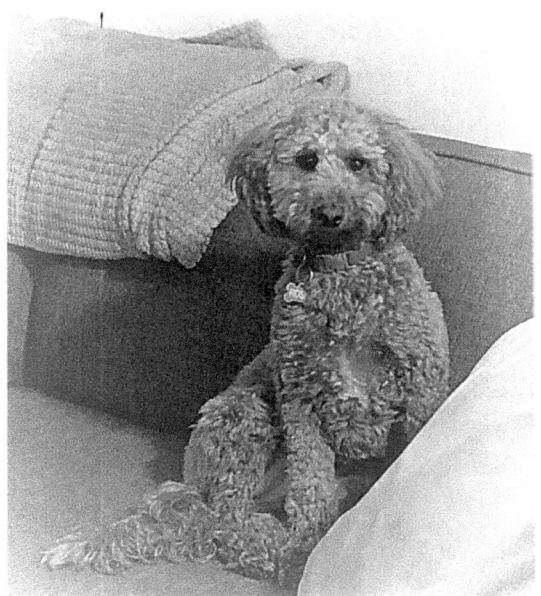

Rosie

The third chakra is also about the emotion of confidence being in balance. Aggression issues show that something is out of balance.

In Chapter 4 you learned about Cato, the dog with aggression issues toward his guardian and how it relaxed and calmed Cato when his guardian grounded and relaxed.

Here is the rest of Cato's story.

The next thing I did was assess Cato. Cato was calm until I got to his third chakra, then he got edgy and was very agitated. Some energy was blocked in his third chakra that was causing his aggressive behavior. Once I cleared and balanced his third chakra, he was calm and confident.

The report afterward from Cato's guardian: he was his old Cato self, and his aggression was gone.

Cato's guardian was thrilled and could relax now with Cato.

CHAPTER 8

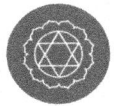

Heart Chakra

THE FOURTH CHAKRA IS CALLED THE HEART CHAKRA.

This chakra is important because it is the center of compassion and joy. It connects all living beings as it is the universal language of love. The third chakra is the bond between the human (guardian) and their pet. Your pet knows and senses your love and connects on the heart level.

This chakra is also a bridge for the lower chakras and the upper chakras. The lower three chakras that we've already discussed are associated with the three-dimensional Earth plane: the physical chakras. The heart chakra bridges the chakras, going up into the higher frequencies of the fifth, sixth, and seventh chakras, considered the spiritual chakras. The heart chakra is the bridge that allows that connection between the physical and the spiritual realms.

The powerful thing about the heart chakra is that it also bridges people and animals, as well as people and people of all nationalities and all languages. The heart chakra is universal.

Color: Green and pink (green for physical/healing, pink for spiritual/love)

Sound: Wam (pronounced Wahm)

Music note: F

Healing Your Animal Essence(s): Chakra 4, love, joy

Emotions: Joy, compassion, sadness, grief

Organs/glands: Heart, pericardium, lungs, cardiac plexus, pulmonary plexus, thymus

Parts of the body: Circulation, cardiovascular system, thoracic spine, upper back, shoulders, forelimbs, chest

Location:

- Back: between the shoulders

- Front: center of the chest

In balance: Your pet is open, friendly, and is connecting with you and other humans and animals. The heart and lungs are healthy.

Out of balance: Your pet may display moping, sadness, anxiety, or act needy. They may have heart or respiratory issues including asthma. Other signs are stroke, hypertension, blood disorders, and arthritis.

Your pet connects and communicates a lot with his/her heart chakra, as other animals do.

A great heart chakra example is when I was in New York City in April 2022, as my business was being featured in the lights on Broadway in the middle of Times Square! It was a very fun experience.

I'm sharing my photo here, showing the joy of celebration. This is the fun side of the heart chakra.

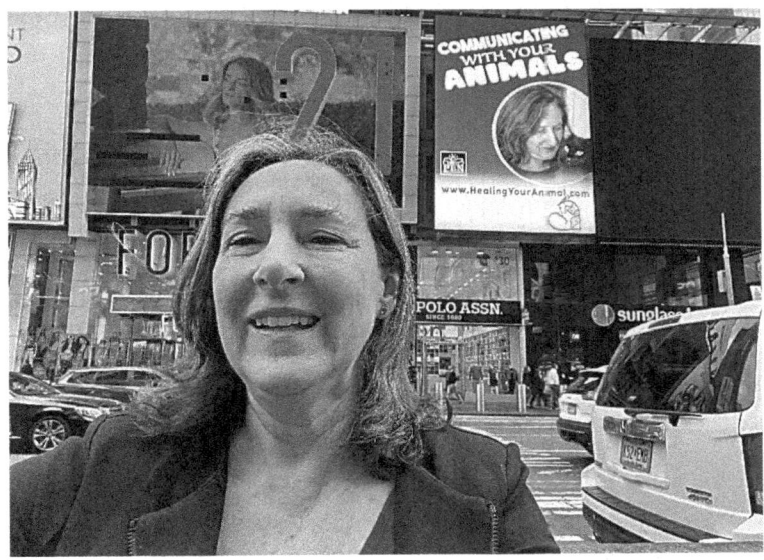

Vicki and Spirit in Times Square

One of the things I had always wanted to do was take a horse and carriage ride in Central Park, so I decided to do it.

Me being me, and my connection with animals, I introduced myself to the horse, named Lucky Sam, with a heart connection. He was eating but stopped mid-chew and looked at me with this "Oh my gosh, you're actually acknowledging me" expression. He was so surprised because people generally are not in that space of connecting with him on the same level. He realized, "Wow, you really are listening to me. You really are connected." That was a fun and memorable heart connection.

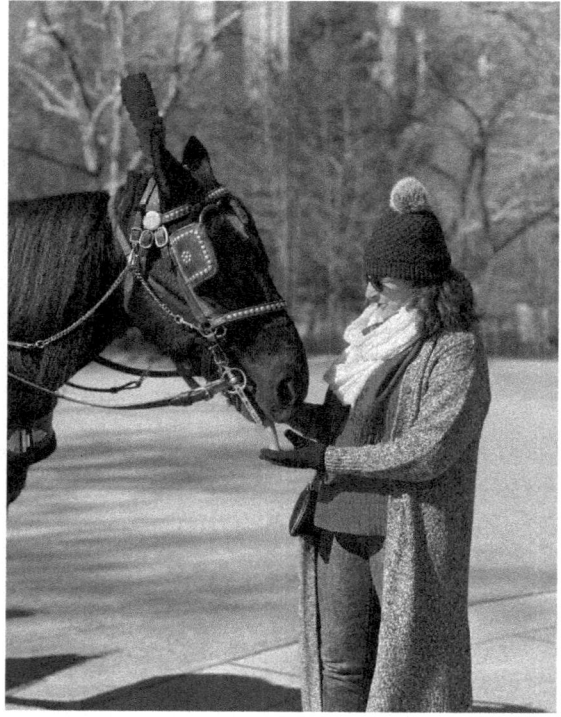

Vicki and Lucky Sam

Animals respond greatly to the heart chakra. If you feel joy and excitement, your pet will get energized and excited with you.

Your pet is sensitive to you, their guardian. If you are sad and grieving, your pet feels this and takes it in. Your pet also feels grief. Where there is a loss, they feel their grief and they feel their guardian's grief.

If you are nervous, unsettled, and anxious, your pet will pick up on this and respond with nervousness and unsettled, hyper behavior.

How Your Heart Chakra Becomes Out of Balance

The heart chakra is all about unconditional love, joy, and compassion. If you have suffered the loss of a loved one, your heart chakra is going to be out of balance due to grief. If you have a lot of sadness and you aren't doing your heart's desires, your heart chakra is out of balance.

How Your Pet's Heart Chakra Becomes Out of Balance

- Their person is feeling grief.
- They have lost their parent/guardian or loved one.
- They have a heart issue.
- They have a respiratory issue.
- They have a blood disorder.
- They have been neglected.
- They aren't fulfilling their purpose.
- They aren't being appreciated for fulfilling their purpose.
- They aren't having play time and connection.

Heart Chakra Dog

Candy is a Bouvier dog that I have known since she was a puppy. I met her when she was just a few days old. Candy is a helper dog. Her guardian, Lynn, took her niece, Alexis, in to live with her when her niece was eight, shortly after Candy was born. Candy became Alexis's dog and support system.

Candy went with Alexis to 4H, where she attended meetings, helping other children learn about dogs. Candy has also been my demonstration dog for multiple presentations, along with being a model for massage, Reiki, and animal communication classes.

Candy's heart chakra has been helping many people throughout her life.

What is consistent with Candy is when she is receiving a healing session, she always almost immediately rolls on her back for me to work her heart chakra.

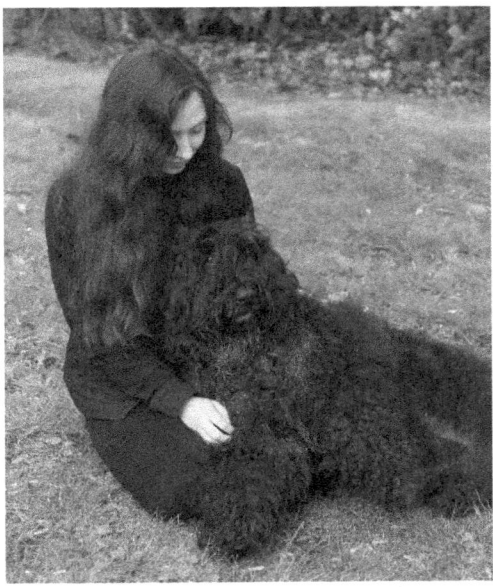

Alexis and Candy

Bouncy to Calm

Min, a Bouvier dog, has a special place in my heart because I was there to assist when she was born.

I was preparing to do a calming demonstration video with Min, who was very bouncy and excited. I had the camera on the stand ready to shoot her video and had a blanket to define a boundary of where she should be. Before I could get the camera rolling, Min came bouncing along, knocking over the stand with the camera on it, getting the microphone cords twisted and causing all kinds of chaos. Too bad I didn't get to capture that on video to show what she was like before calming her by balancing her heart chakra.

Min and I got on the blanket. Lynn, Min's guardian, got the video rolling, and Min calmed down quickly with the heart chakra balancing.

The heart chakra is the center of the chest. There is an acupressure point called CV17 in the center of the chest. It is one of the most calming points on the body, so balancing the heart chakra includes stimulating (and calming) the body.

Min is a good example of how a dog that is revved up can mellow very quickly by balancing the heart chakra. With some dogs, you have to breathe slowly and hold the heart chakra patiently while the balancing and calming take effect.

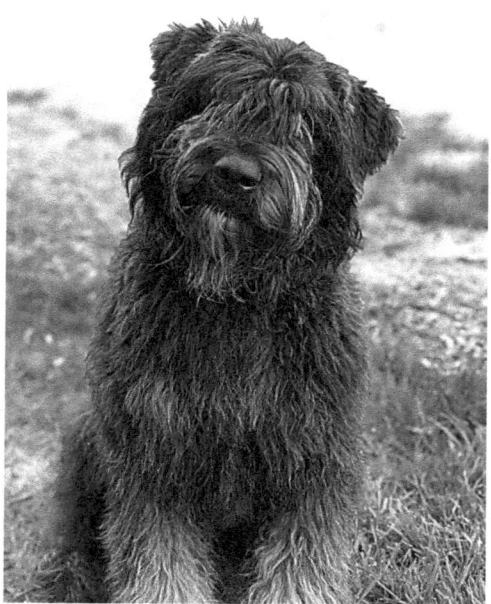

Min

CHAPTER 9

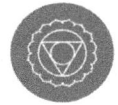

Throat Chakra

THE FIFTH CHAKRA IS CALLED THROAT CHAKRA.

This chakra is important because it is about self-expression.

Color: Sky blue

Sound: Ham (pronounced Hahm)

Musical note: G

Healing Your Animal Essence: Chakra 5, voice

Emotions: Expressive, repression

Organs/glands: Large intestine, laryngeal plexus, lungs, thyroid

Parts of the body: Neck, throat, esophagus, jaw, mouth, teeth, tongue, lips, nose, ears, cervical ganglia, medulla plexus

Location:

- Back: back of the neck

- Front: center of the neck

In balance: Healthy communication and expression, with barks and meows. Healthy thyroid, swallowing, and teeth.

Out of balance: Excessive meowing, excessive barking, or the inability to meow or bark or a very low, strained sound. Thyroid issues, bad breath, or trouble swallowing. The neck may be out of balance, or animals may carry their head low.

The throat is the center for expression of voice. Sometimes the expression is coming from an imbalance in another chakra, such as stress barking and aggressive hissing or growling. The throat chakra will need balancing as it is being overworked. When balancing the throat chakra, it is important to remember to balance the rest of the chakras too.

How Your Throat Chakra Becomes Out of Balance

The throat chakra is all about authentic self-expression and communication. If you are holding back words, afraid to speak up, or expressing words with no filters, not listening, choking, or have a sore throat, your throat chakra is out of balance.

How Your Pet's Throat Chakra Becomes Out of Balance

- Their person has an imbalanced throat chakra.

- They demonstrate excessive meowing/barking.

- They have been stifled from barking, such as with a shock collar.

- They have thyroid issues.

- They have a stiff neck or shoulders.

- They have ear issues.

New Apartment Caused Stress Barking

Rosie, a mini Goldendoodle, had been stress-barking all day while her guardian was at work. They had just moved, and Rosie was not used to her new apartment and all the noises. I was balancing Rosie's throat chakra, and it was very soothing to her throat. Rosie also received full-body chakra balancing to help where she was out of balance in multiple chakras with separation anxiety, not feeling safe in a new place, and not having a good appetite.

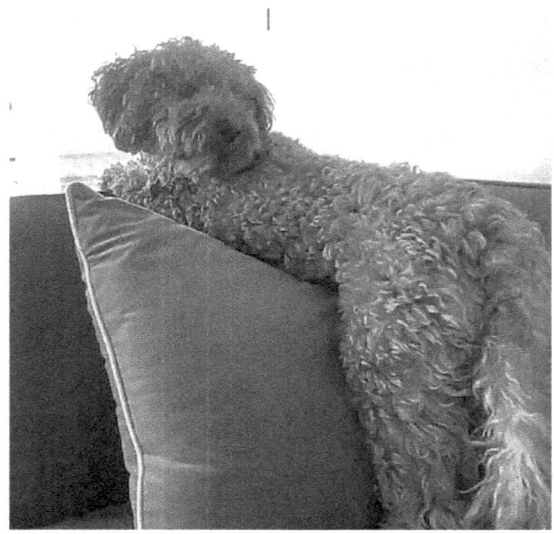

Rosie

Cat Requests Throat Chakra Support

Miguel and Diana were going out of town and wanted an animal communication session to make sure that their cat companion, Nirvana, understood what was happening. They wanted to discuss when they would be gone, when they would be back, and who was taking care of her while they were gone. During our session, Nirvana asked me to balance her throat chakra. She was content having her throat chakra supported. When I mentioned this to Diana, she said that Nirvana has an overactive thyroid. As mentioned above, the thyroid is part of the throat chakra.

Nirvana knew the support she wanted and asked for it.

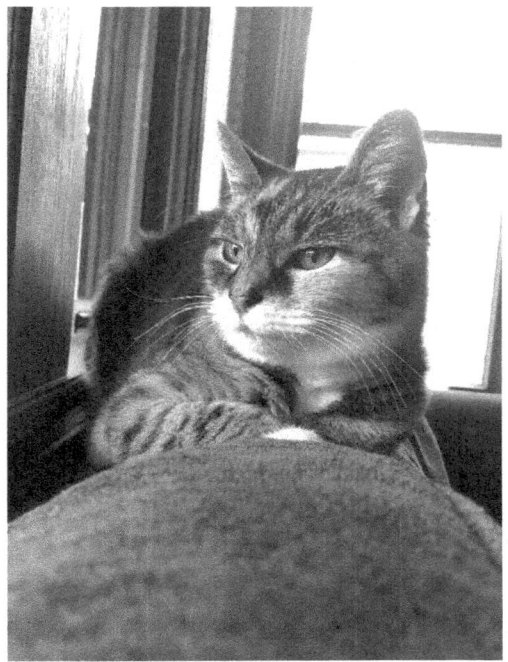

Nirvana

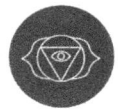

CHAPTER 10

Third Eye Chakra

THE SIXTH CHAKRA IS CALLED THIRD EYE CHAKRA and is also known as the brow chakra. This chakra is important as it is about intuition, clear seeing, imagination, and mental clarity.

Color: Indigo blue

Sound: Om (pronounced Ohm)

Musical note: A

Healing Your Animal Essence: Chakra 6, Om

Emotions: Clarity, detachment

Organs/glands: Gallbladder, cavernous plexus, small intestine, pituitary gland

Parts of the body: Mind, lower brain, mid forehead, back of head, eyes, central nervous system, hypothalamus, pituitary plexus, upper sinus, temples, triple warmer

Location:

- Back: back of the head

- Front: center of the forehead

In balance: Animals think and see clearly. Their eyes are bright and engaging.

Out of balance: Animals may be easily confused or display a lack of focus, not picking up training quickly. Eye issues and sinus issues may appear.

How Your Third Eye Chakra Becomes Out of Balance

This chakra is important as it is about intuition, clear seeing, imagination, telepathy, visualization, and mental clarity. If you have trouble focusing, feel disconnected, are unable to rise out of details and see big picture, have a headache or eye issues, your third eye chakra is out of balance.

How Your Pet's Third Eye Chakra Becomes Out of Balance

- Their person's third eye chakra is out of balance.

- They have trouble focusing.

- They have dull eyes.

- They seem confused.

- They have a headache.

- They have eye issues.

- They have a brain tumor.

Yes, cats and dogs get headaches. You may notice a furrowed brow, being sullen, or they may hide due to being sensitive to noise and lights.

Headaches in Pets

Early on in my career, I had an in-person session with Jake, a mixed-breed dog, whose guardians wanted to help him feel his best. Jake and I were on the floor on the big dog bed together. His guardians were on the couch watching. Looking at Jake's face, I noticed his eyes were sullen and his face was furrowed at the brow. I mentioned to his guardians that Jake had a headache. They were surprised to hear this, as they didn't know dogs could get headaches. This stood out to me because it was so evident to me, and it was so foreign to his guardians. By the end of Jake's session, his face was relaxed, and his eyes were beaming brightly. It was obvious that Jake was feeling much better.

Cat Gets Headache from Guardian

Spirit, my black domestic long-hair cat, is very connected with me. I had a sinus infection that really knocked me down, and Spirit was right by my side. I noticed he was starting to have trouble focusing, and he was not as alert as usual. He wasn't quite himself.

He seemed confused when he was playing with his toy, not as quick as normal and not tracking it well. I then got an intuitive flash, realizing he was helping me clear my sinus issues, and it was affecting him.

When I cleared and balanced his sixth chakra, he was bright-eyed, alert, and it was evident he was feeling better. He was back happily and eagerly playing with his toy. He was fully alert, tracking the toy, and pouncing with great precision.

Since my sinus issue was a process that took a while to heal, Spirit would keep helping me clear my sinus issues, and it kept affecting him. Clearing and balancing Spirit's chakra energy regularly kept Spirit living his best playful, alert, interactive, and affectionate self.

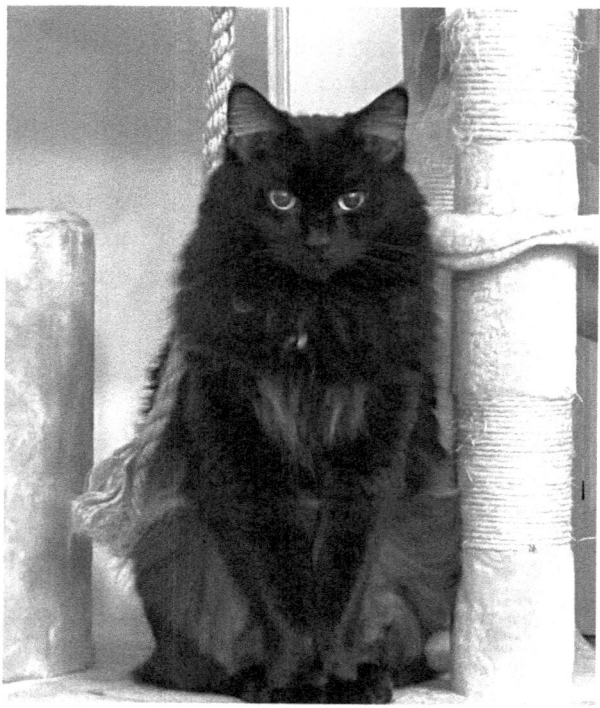

Spirit

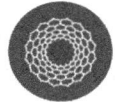

CHAPTER 11

Crown Chakra

THE SEVENTH CHAKRA IS CALLED THE CROWN CHAKRA.

This chakra is important as it is our connection to the Divine, Universe, God, Spirit, Higher Power, whatever term is meaningful to you. To your pet it comes naturally as it is the crown chakra that connects with the highest form of wisdom and intelligence in their world.

Color: Purple or may contain white ard gold

Sound: Aum (pronounced Ahm)

Musical note: B

Healing Your Animal Essence: Chakra 7, enlightenment

Emotions: Cosmic consciousness, worry, depression

Organs/glands: pineal gland, liver, gallbladder, bladder, Governing Vessel

Governing Vessel (GV) is a meridian in TCM (traditional Chinese medicine) called the "Sea of Yang Meridians." The GV meridian is a series of 28 acupuncture points running from the base of the spine, up the back, over the head, and ending inside the mouth. It is connected to all yang meridians and thereby governs the energy of the body and supplies energy to deficient meridians, organs, or body parts.

Parts of the body: Top of head, cerebral cortex, pineal plexus, central nervous system, fur/hair, upper brain, spine

Location: Top of the head in the center, in front of the bump (external occipital protuberance)

In balance: Animal is alert, spirited, engaging, and happy.

Out of balance: An animal may seem disconnected, distant, not fitting into playing with others. Other signs are seizures, being overly sensitive to influences in the environment, dementia, senility (in cats this is called feline cognitive dysfunction, and in dogs it is called canine cognitive dysfunction or Alzheimer's disease). Physical ailments may appear such as epilepsy, multiple sclerosis (MS) (for dogs it is called degenerative myelopathy [DM]), or migraines.

How Your Crown Chakra Becomes Out of Balance

The crown chakra is all about divine connection to Source, oneness with all that is, wisdom, spirituality. It's the place where selfless service comes in; it's above the ego. If you are feeling a sense of separation from Source, such as panic attacks, depression, dementia, post-traumatic stress disorder, multiple sclerosis, or seizures, your crown chakra is out of balance.

How Your Pet's Crown Chakra Becomes Out of Balance

- Their person is dealing with panic attacks, depression, dementia, post-traumatic stress disorder, multiple sclerosis, or seizures.

- They are experiencing seizures.

- They have experienced trauma.

- They experience the death or loss of their guardian.

- They are feeling devastated by being rehomed or moved.

- They are shut down from the world.

Having Seizures

Finn, a nine-year-old cat, was adopted into his new forever home. He was on seizure medication to control his seizures but still having seizures on a regular basis.

Finn was being less interactive, less affectionate, and had lost interest in play time. He had also gotten irritable with being brushed when he enjoyed it before.

Nancy, Finn's guardian, contacted me to support Finn reducing his seizures and adjusting to his new forever home, where Finn would be happier, more affectionate, more playful, and enjoy his brushing again.

Finn responded well to his chakra balancing sessions. Each session was going deeper into healing layers in Finn's body and allowing Finn's body's self-healing mechanism to get a boost taking over healing. This allowed Finn to be his healthiest self. The seizures decreased in frequency and duration between each session.

In Finn's session, he communicated where he wanted his scratching post and water fountain as he wasn't using them where they were currently placed. Here's the report I received back:

"After Finn's session yesterday, we moved the scratching post his previous owners gave us. Moved it next to the dining table and by evening, Finn used it twice and early this morning! Never would have crossed our minds to place it there, but he's happy, so we're happy. :) Also moved things away from the wall where his fountain is and pulled the fountain further away from the wall. Finn began drinking from his water fountain daily. He likes the extra space around his fountain. :) He no longer wants to drink from the bathtub faucet. His appetite for wet food seems to have increased a bit, yet he doesn't overeat. Continues to use his scratching post almost daily. Thanks again for all your help with Finn!"

—Nancy, Seattle, Washington

Playing and Bumping Head

Niles, a domestic shorthair cat, is a regular monthly client that I meet with by video. This means that I know Niles, so when something is not his normal, I recognize it. Brenda, one of Nile's guardians, reached out to see if Niles could get an additional session as he was moping, lethargic, not eating, and not interested in playing. She was concerned. In this session, Nile's crown chakra was blocked. This was unusual for him. In talking with Brenda, I discovered that Niles had been playing hard and had skidded into the wall a couple of times, bumping his head. As his crown chakra was opening, Niles started responding and perking up. He continued perking up and was clear-headed and alert when his seventh chakra became fully balanced. After Niles received his full chakra balancing session, he started eating and playing and was back to his normal kitty self.

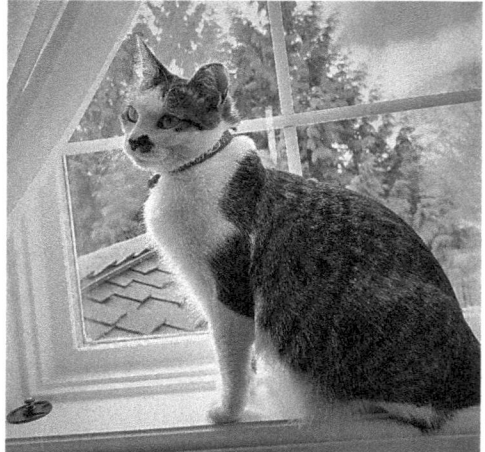

Niles

CHAPTER 12

Rescue Rehabilitation

RESCUE ANIMALS WILL HAVE AN UNBALANCED ROOT CHAKRA because they are not or were not in their forever home. They feel this and know this, no matter how good the temporary situation is for them. And when they come to you, even though you know it is your pet's forever home, they do not.

Fears and unmet needs go into the root chakra and then move up the chain to all the other chakras. These fears are fed into the nervous system. This explains why pets (and people) with a rough beginning generally have more trouble calming and feeling settled than others. It takes effort and patience to support and heal the balancing of the pet for a stable, calming effect.

This is one of my specialties. And it is so rewarding when an animal (or person) has the pivotal shift of switching from operating in the sympathetic nervous system (fight or flight) to the parasympathetic nervous system, being in a calmer place.

The stories in this section revolve around cats that were cared for with the Feral Care Sanctuary, located at the Whole Cat and Kaboodle pet store and cat café.

QR Code: 3D Viewing of Vicki Doing a Healing Session with Cat Opie in the Whole Cat and Kaboodle Cat Cafe

Chakra 1 (Root)

Peg, a calico cat, was surrendered into Nancy's care at the Feral Cat Sanctuary because there was a young child at home that was causing Peg anxiety. Peg was stressed, shut down, had a poor appetite, and wouldn't come out of her cubby. I was called in to see if I could calm her and get her to eat. When I greeted her, her eyes were big and wide—she was on alert. Her body was tense. Even though she was scared, she let me put my hand in the cubby to work with her. She had a lot of imbalances in her root chakra. There was heat coming off her low back. Heat in an area means energy is collected there that isn't flowing to the rest of the body. In my experience, it is associated with inflammation and probable discomfort. The heat dissipated as the chakra came back into balance. Peg also had a lot of energy imbalances in her sixth chakra, around her face. I balanced all her chakras. By the end of Peg's session, she was lying peacefully, with eyes shut and face relaxed. I recommended a follow-up as there was more to release and she had done all she could for this session.

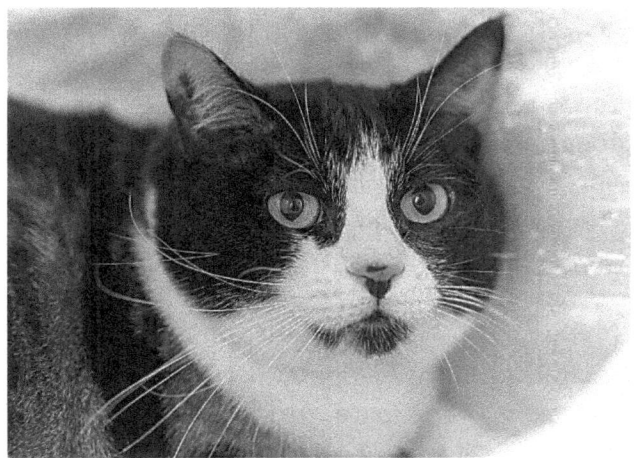

Peg

During the next session, she was in her cubby. She started walking toward me, putting her front legs out of her cubby as if she wanted to come all the way out, yet she couldn't quite bring herself to do it. This was a big shift—attempting to come out. We were in an open area, and she was on alert when there was a person or movement nearby. While balancing her root chakra, she was getting more and more comfortable, and she was being less reactive to people and movements. She was still staying in her cubby.

For her next session, I brought her in her cubby to a private office. I wanted her to feel safe. She was responding and getting calmer. I lifted the cubby and encouraged her to come out. She was afraid at first. I was working at a distance to help her as she sat under the chair. She got more comfortable and started exploring the office more confidently. This was a big step for her! I opened up the cubby so she could go back in because I had promised if she came out, she could go back in. A balanced root chakra is very important for your pet to feel safe. As you can see with Peg, it does make a difference.

Meeko is a cat brought into Nancy at the Feral Cat Sanctuary after his guardian died. He was so distressed. Pacing, hissing, growling; no one could get near him in his kennel. He was very fractious when he met me, hissing, growling, wide-eyed on alert and very unsettled, so I worked with him from a distance. The first thing I did was introduce myself and tell him that I was there to help. Then I started with the root chakra to help with taking the edge off being in a new situation with new people and not understanding why. I started explaining to Meeko where he was and why. He was willing to listen and participate, taking in the chakra healing energy and allowing it to support him. I then worked my way up his chakras. His heart chakra needed extra support as there was grief there to release. Meeko was missing his guardian. Once his heart chakra got relief, Meeko started settling. He shifted from unsettled to laying down, softening his eyes, and then closing them while I finished balancing his chakras. After this session, Meeko made a big shift to roaming the cat café and being adopted to his new forever home.

Animals don't have the placebo effect. Everything is real for them. By opening to receiving the support, Meeko is a great teacher, showing the power of energy healing and communication and the difference it made in his life. I am so proud of him.

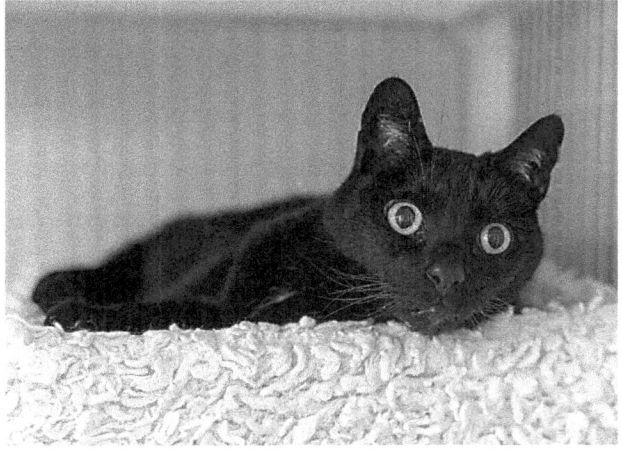

Meeko

Chakra 2 (Sacral)

Early on in my career, I volunteered at the Humane Society doing healing sessions on dogs that needed a boost to get them ready for adoption. One puppy named Michelle was frozen in fear. She couldn't walk due to being so scared. I started with the root chakra to help release some fear and continued up the chakras. The sacral chakra needed balancing. Her muscles and body were tense and taut in this area. The importance of this area was that she was getting spayed in the next few days. It was good timing for my healing session with her. Having her sacral chakra more relaxed and balanced prepared her for her spay surgery for an easier time with recovery. When I showed up the next week for my volunteer healing work, I was hoping to do a post-surgery check on her, yet I didn't get to. Michelle was already adopted. I was so grateful for the timing of her healing support we had together. I shudder at the thought of what she would have gone through without the healing support before her surgery being as tight and frozen in fear as she was when I first met her.

For males, it's also helpful before and after neutering to balance sacral chakra.

Chakra 3 (Solar Plexus)

Pumba, a black domestic shorthair cat, was overweight and had a heart murmur. His guardian wanted euthanasia. Luckily, he was released into Nancy's care at the sanctuary. He was hiding and wouldn't eat much, so Nancy asked for my support.

What I found was that Pumba had a block in his digestive area and a block in his throat chakra, No wonder he didn't want to eat! Both chakras opened and cleared. His energy flow was good now, but his physical body was weak due to not eating. I recommended a follow-up session, as blocked and depleted as he was.

When I arrived, I was shown this cute picture of Pumba where he was out in the café thinking he was hiding behind the lamp.

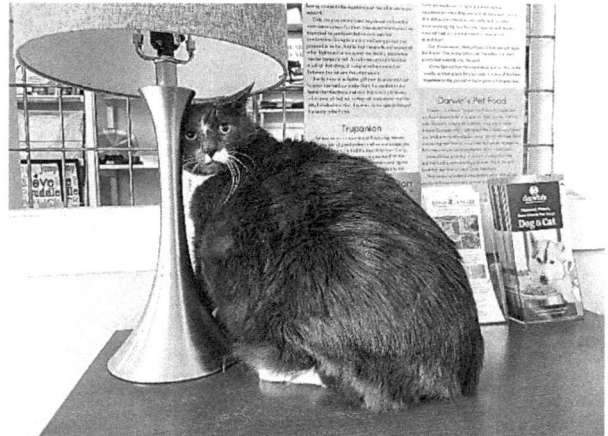

Pumba Hiding Behind a Lamp

At Pumba's follow-up session, he was excited to greet me; it comforted him to see me. Starting out, I discovered his previous chakra balancing had held, the digestive area (chakra 3) and throat (chakra 5) were still open and flowing. We went deeper in this session. I gave him continued support for his digestion/appetite, throat chakra, feeling safe, kidneys, liver, and all his organs. By the end he was showing me telepathically a visual of him happily running around, so I felt good about his progress. When an animal shows me something, I know it is going to happen because it is coming from them.

Later, when I checked in to ask about Pumba, I found out Pumba is now living it up, being a big ham in his new forever home. I am so happy for him.

Chakra 4 (Heart)

Marley is an obese black domestic shorthair cat. He is a real sweetheart. Marley and his sister were found at an estate sale after their guardians had died. They were brought into Nancy's care at the sanctuary. Marley was shut down, frozen in grief with the shock of his situation. I was called in because nothing was getting through to him, and he needed to eat soon or he was going to die. I went to work. I connected with him, supporting him with healing to loosen his grip from fear, stimulate his appetite, and relieve the pain of his grief so he could be open to his new situation and begin to trust.

He communicated that he was worried about his sister, so I also did a session with her. I was doing what it took to help Marley feel calm and settled in his new surroundings.

There was still something he wasn't letting go of emotionally.

He ended up in the emergency veterinary clinic. He wasn't eating, his body was struggling, and they were talking about euthanasia as the humane thing to do. I was connecting with him remotely to support him while he was at the veterinary clinic. I hadn't given up on him. Marley's bond with his guardian was so strong and his grief was so deep that I wasn't sure how to get through to him. Then I realized, and he confirmed, that he was hoping to be with his guardian on the other side. I shared that he could live and still connect with her in spiritual form. He liked this. That was the shift he needed. He knew he had to eat to stay alive or he could choose not to eat and die. He chose to eat and rebounded back to life.

Marley's story demonstrates the power of a heartache on the heart chakra. You can see how the other chakras were affected as well. His physical body was under duress until he cleared his emotional issue.

Marley is a great example of how medical care and alternative care work together. You need both for well-rounded care.

Thank you, Marley, for your wonderful, big heart that is helping us learn the depths of heart connections between pets and their guardians and choosing to trust and live again.

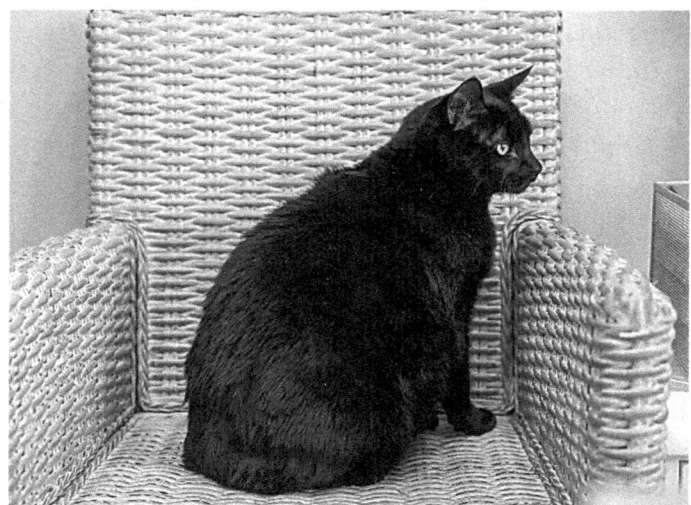

Marley

Chakra 5 (Throat)

Cassidy was surrendered to Nancy's sanctuary a few years ago. Approximately 12 years old, Cassie is a domestic shorthair tortie cat that lives with Nancy now. Cassidy had been diagnosed with hyperthyroidism, which is being managed. She is a very sweet and friendly cat.

Cassidy was having issues with one of Nancy's other cats, Turtle Dove, and was attacking her. This had Nancy believing Cassidy had some problems.

The initial energy scan overall seemed as if Cassidy was struggling and not feeling her best. I found congestion in Cassidy's throat chakra. She started releasing some hissy, angry energy right away.

Being empathic, I could feel Cassidy's sadness she was carrying in her heart chakra. This is where I check my grounding and stay grounded so I can best support her as she releases it.

Cassidy's sacral chakra received support with a tune-up for her kidneys. It is common in older cats for their kidneys to need a boost.

In Cassidy's root chakra, she had some irritableness, a lot of anger, and grumpiness flying out of her body that needed to be released to help her heal. This felt as if it was from being displaced, rehomed, or something from her past.

Following the energy in Cassidy's body and what energy she needed to release, I could sense that she needed an overall chakra balancing from the top down vs. the bottom up.

After her root chakra balanced, the throat chakra showed up again for another layer of healing where gagging energy was purging.

At this point, all of Cassidy's energy was flowing smoothly from the root chakra (base of tail) all the way up through the rest of the chakras up to the crown chakra (top of head).

When there are deep-seated issues with animals, they don't always clear the multiple layers on the first session. This is especially true for humans. The longer the issue has been going on, the longer it takes to heal.

Animals will clear issues quicker than humans. With humans, we have to clear the mental as well as the cellular levels. With animals, they only have to clear issues out of the cellular level. Animals don't have an ego.

When there are deep-seated issues with animals, I recommend a three-session series to get to the core and stabilize the issue/situation.

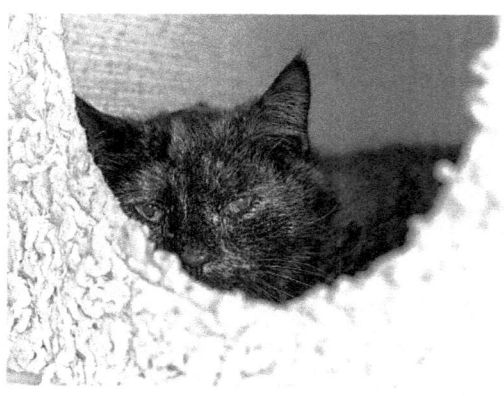

Cassidy

Chakra 6 (Third Eye)

Cheerio, a black domestic shorthair cat, had hyperthyroidism that his guardian didn't treat. Cheerio was howling a lot, which is why his guardian released him into Nancy's care. The untreated hyperthyroidism caused Cheerio to have high blood pressure, which caused Cheerio to go blind. Under Nancy's care, Cheerio was put on appropriate medications. I was asked to support him and balance his body because he wasn't eating much since he had these issues going on. He had his favorite spot where I worked with him.

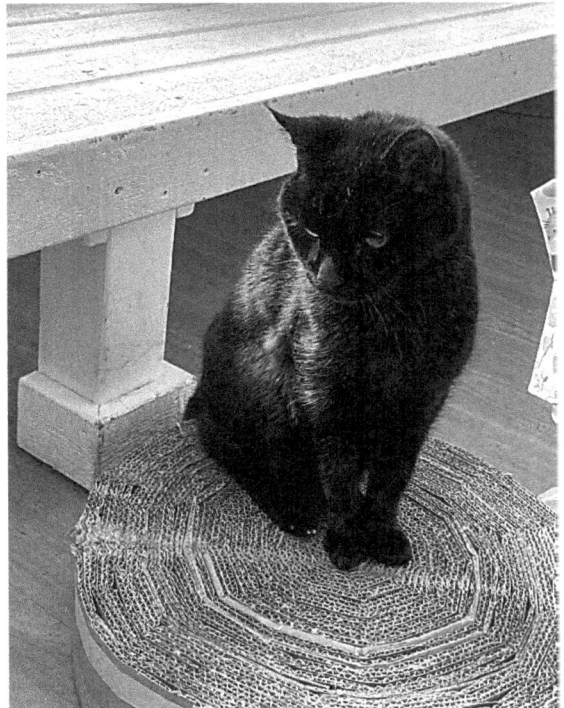
Cheerio on Cardboard Cat Scratcher

In his session, Cheerio needed an overall balancing. I balanced all of his chakras. He also needed a little massage to get him feeling better. You can find out more about using massage in my book *Heart to Heart: How you can heal your animal through all stages of life*.

When I was balancing his sixth chakra, there was crackling energy happening around his eyes. I had not felt that before. I could feel the healing energy supporting his eyesight coming back.

After this session, Cheerio rebounded very nicely, eating and gaining some eyesight back. He isn't using his whiskers to sense his surroundings like he was having to do initially. He is now the store cat at Whole Cat and Kaboodle. You'll find him lounging around, greeting customers, and sometimes sporting a Spiderman suit.

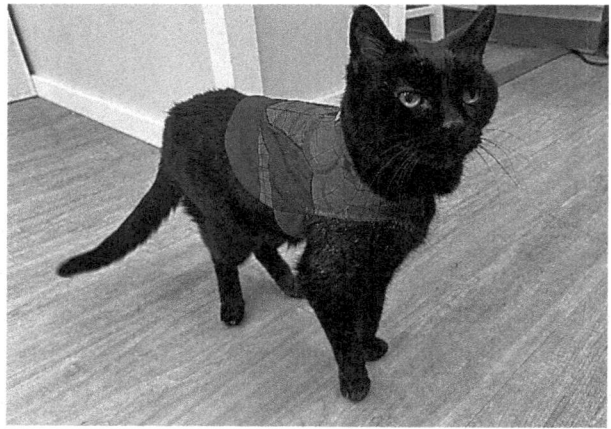

Cheerio Sporting his Spiderman Suit

Chakra 7 (Crown)

Four-year-old Jack the cat had been surrendered to The Whole Cat and Kaboodle from his guardian, who was unable to take care of herself and therefore, unable to take care of Jack. Jack was living in unsanitary, hoarder-like conditions due to the decline of his guardian's health.

He came to the right place. The Whole Cat and Kaboodle staff take good care of the cats there.

Jack was being force-bottle-fed to get nourishment in him.

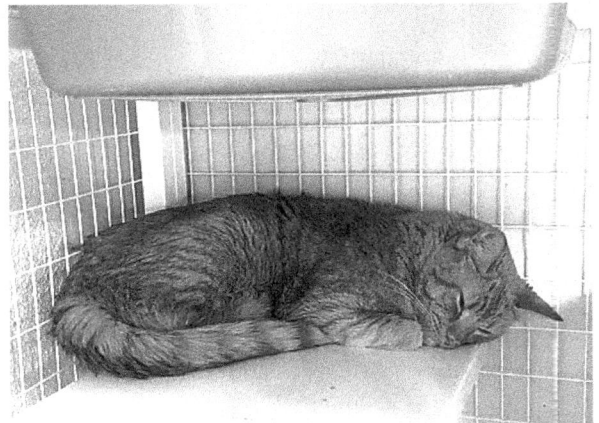

Jack, Emotionally Shut Down, Having to be Bottle-Fed

They called me in to see if Jack wanted to live and what he desired.

He was disconnected, very shut down, and initially not very responsive. His crown chakra was blocked, and I was concerned.

Then Jack started responding to the seventh chakra balancing. Once that opened, he received full-body balancing.

He started eating on his own.

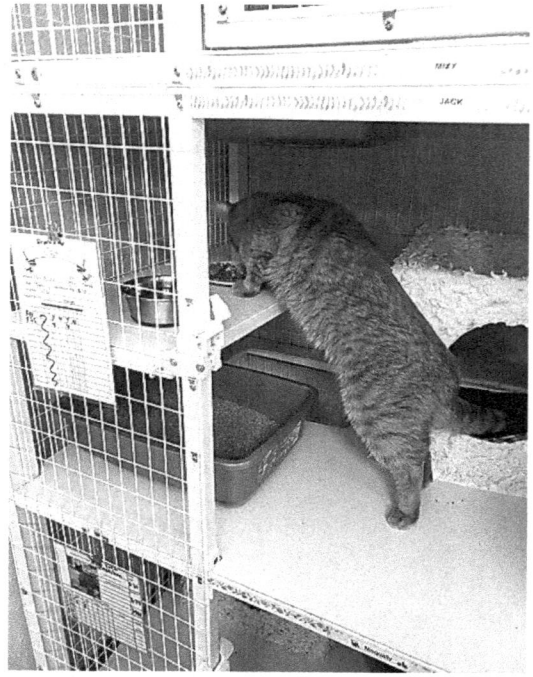

Jack Up and Eating on His Own After Chakra Balancing

Then Jack became curious, walking around and engaging with the staff. He became playful. And today, he has a forever home.

It was so rewarding to watch his transformation and to be a part of helping him live his best life.

CHAPTER 13

Preparing You

NOW YOU ARE READY TO BEGIN the process of working with your pet's chakras.

The first step is to make sure you are grounded, present, and in a calm state of mind before connecting with and starting to work with your pet.

It's important to understand what affects your sense of safety and calm in your life and how you can support yourself in shifting from stress and out of sorts to calm and present. (The scientific name for this is shifting out of fight-or-flight mode or sympathetic nervous system, to being in your parasympathetic nervous system.)

This is especially important if you have a rescue pet or a pet that is high energy. They will highly benefit from you being in a calm space.

The more grounded you are, the more grounded and calm your pet will be.

Pets feed off their environment. If you, the pet parent, are not firmly rooted (grounded), your pet is going to be off on some level, and their behavior may escalate. Some pets are more grounded than others naturally so their behaviors won't be as escalated and off the charts; however, they will be unsettled.

The root chakra is all about the sense of safety and survival. If you're not feeling safe and secure, your root chakra is going to be out of balance. If you're not stable in your finances, food, and shelter, your root chakra is out of balance, and your pet's root chakra will be out of balance. They look to you for this safety and security.

It is important to balance and keep balancing your root chakra because the rest of your chakras depend on the root chakra being stable. Keeping a balanced chakra system helps you be in your best health.

Things That Affect Your Root Chakra Getting Out of Balance

- You are not feeling safe.
- You have health issues.
- Your loved ones have health issues.
- You are experiencing money problems.
- You are experiencing job stress.
- You are stressed about traffic.
- You are preparing for travel.
- You are moving.
- You have a new relationship or marriage.

- You are going through a breakup or divorce.
- You are grieving the death of a loved one.
- You have a new baby/child/person coming into family.
- You have a new pet coming into family.
- A child is moving out or going off to college.
- It is a holiday or holiday season.
- You are having company over.
- You are experiencing a natural disaster.

You have heard me talk about grounding. Let's dive in and learn how.

Ground Yourself Before Working with Your Animal

We are going to start with grounding you first. Because anytime you are going to go work with any animal or person, you want to ground first. If you are not stable and grounded, the animal or person you are working with is going to feel your ungroundedness. It will not feel soothing to them. If you are not grounded and focused with an animal, they will be unsettled and most likely walk away.

I recommend that you make a recording of this grounding exercise with your own voice reading it before you start. You can listen to the recording or have someone read this exercise to you so you can close your eyes, go inward, and benefit with the full experience of this exercise.

Grounding Exercise

Sit or stand and feel your feet touching the floor beneath you. Take a moment and close your eyes. If you are not at a place where you can close your eyes, pretend or imagine you can.

Take a moment and check in with how you are feeling at this moment. What is going on in your body? What is going on in your head? Are you feeling disconnected or scattered? Are you feeling centered and clear? No judgment, just notice. Do you feel floaty? Do you feel heavy energetically? Again, no judgment, just notice.

Now, pay attention to your feet. Take a moment to feel a very solid connection with the floor. I invite you to begin moving, rocking forward and backward on your feet while standing on the floor. Raise up your heels and stand on the balls of your feet. Now lower your heels and raise your toes up in the air while resting on the heels of your feet. Do this a couple more times back and forth, to really get a good feel of your feet connecting with the floor. Repeat this a few times. And as your awareness is going to the ground with your focus on your feet on the floor, take a moment and feel that connection.

Now, feel the connection of your feet resting flat on the floor. Feel the connection of your feet going down through the floor and sensing the Earth underneath. As your feet are connecting to the Earth underneath your floor and you feel the Earth (going through floors between you and the Earth if needed), imagine you have roots coming out of the soles of your feet going down into the Earth as deep as feels comfortable for them. Find the sweet spot for the roots going down into the

Earth. Roots grow vertically into the ground, and they also grow horizontally. Imagine roots are coming out the soles of your feet and then growing horizontally. They are going as wide as they want to. When this feels good, find your grounding cord coming out from the center of your root chakra (base of your spine) and see it going down through the floor, through the Earth, all the way down to the center of the Earth. If you are unsure where your grounding cord is, it comes out of your body at your perineum, which is located between your vagina for females/your scrotum for males and your anus. If you are unable to see or feel this, pretend or imagine you can.

You are taking the end of the cord and pulling it down, all the way down to the center of the Earth. And on your way down to the center of the Earth, imagine putting in some stakes, hooking your cord into the Earth as you go down, so if it comes untethered at the core, you are still down into the Earth and can easily get back down to full grounding. And as your grounding cord is going down and hooking into the Earth and then going down farther and hooking into the Earth and going down farther and hooking into the Earth and continuing all the way down to the center of the Earth, where you can hook in and wrap your grounding cord around the core of the Earth. There is a ball of light, a core of light. So keep going down deep until you reach this light. This light feeds your grounding cord. Now take a moment and feel how this feels. Feel your deep connection with the Earth, your solid connection. Your feet and legs feel grounded, solid, and stable. Now put your attention back on your grounding cord all the way in the center of the Earth, deeply connected to the Earth. You have a tripod of grounding energy support with your legs and grounding cord.

Now you have a knowing—this is what deep grounding is. Take a moment and sense how this feels. Sense how you feel, how your body feels. Sense how deep grounding feels to you.

This is now in your cellular memory. You always have this with you. When you are feeling a little off or ungrounded, you can remember this activation and easily get back to this feeling. Take another moment and really embrace how this feels.

Do you notice a difference in how you feel now from when you started this grounding activation? How so? What is different now? This information will help you. Remember this grounded feeling.

You can open your eyes.

This is what grounded feels like. If you are not feeling this in your day, it is an indication that you need to ground.

The chakras are an ancient known source for health and healing.

Now is the time to start balancing your chakras if you aren't already. You are not only doing this for you; you are also doing it for your pet.

Now that you are grounded, let's balance your chakras.

I recommend that you make a recording of this healing activation with your own voice reading it before you start. You can listen to the recording or have someone read this exercise to you so you can close your eyes, go inward, and benefit with the full experience of balancing your chakras.

Healing Activation: Balancing Your Chakras

When you are preparing to balance your pet's chakras, it is important to balance your chakras first. Here is an exercise to walk you through balancing your chakras.

I invite you to step away from whatever you have been doing in your day and allow your attention to be fully in this moment. Be right here, right now. All that has happened and is yet to happen will be there for you when you get back. Take a moment and gently close your eyes. If you are not at a place where you can physically close your eyes, pretend or imagine you can.

Take a moment and check in with how you feel. No judgment, just check in and see if there are tight, sore, or heavy parts of your body. Check in and see where your body feels good, light, maybe even tingly. Just notice.

I now invite you to take a deep breath in, hold it, let it out. Now take another deep breath in, hold it, let it out. And now for the power of three, take a deep breath in, hold it, and let it out. This allows you to become present and more fully in the moment.

As we are starting our way on this journey:

Chakra 1 is the root chakra. It is located at the base of your spine; its color is red, and it is closest to the earth with the densest frequency. It represents survival and safety.

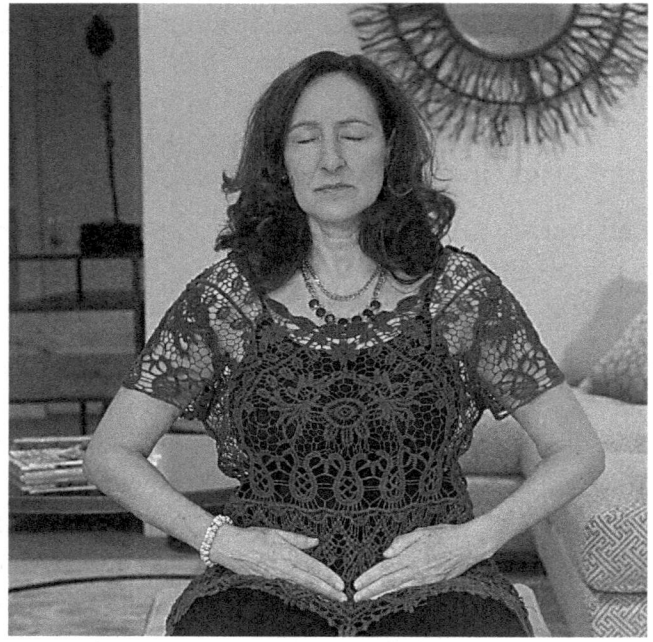

Chakra 1

Place your hands on your lower pelvic region. Imagine your root chakra is cleansing and clearing all that is no longer needed and allowing in the energy of a balanced, healthy root chakra.

Chakra 2 is the sacral chakra. It is located two inches below your navel; its color is orange. This chakra represents your sexuality, the birthing not only of physical children, but also the birthing of new ideas and projects, the center of your creativity and passions.

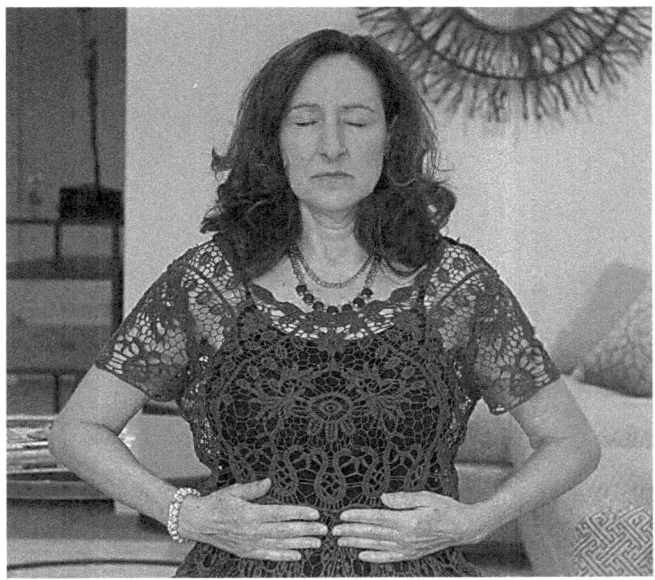

Chakra 2

Place your hands on your lower abdomen two inches below your navel. Imagine your sacral chakra is cleansing and clearing all that is no longer needed and allowing in the energy of a balanced, healthy sacral chakra.

Chakra 3 is the solar plexus chakra. It is located between your belly button and the base of your rib cage; its color is yellow. It is your center of power, your center of will, and how you present yourself to the world. It is also your center of manifestation, so when you state your desires and intentions into the world, they can be answered and delivered to you.

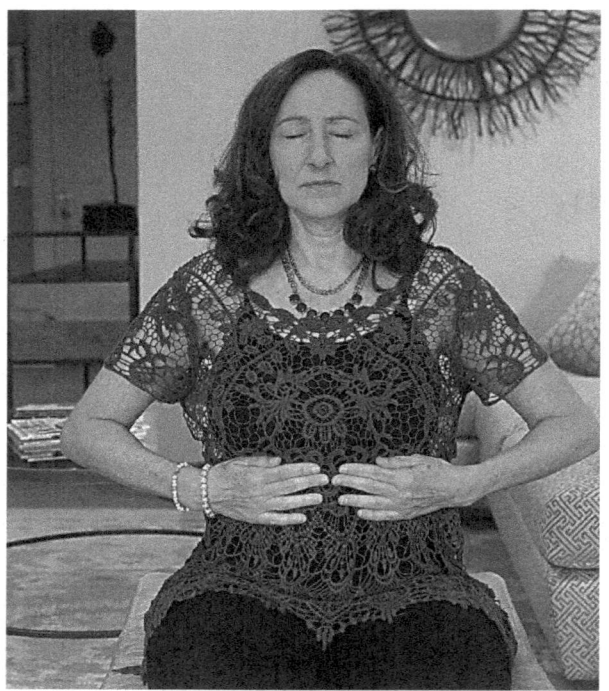

Chakra 3

Place your hands on your abdomen above your navel and below your rib cage. Imagine your solar plexus chakra is cleansing and clearing all that is no longer needed and allowing in the energy of a balanced, healthy solar plexus chakra.

Chakra 4 is the heart chakra. It is located in the center of your chest; its color is green. It is the center of love, unconditional love, and compassion. This is the connection with oneness, with everyone. From your heart, this chakra represents a universal language of love; this goes for your animals too. They know and sense this love and connect on the heart level.

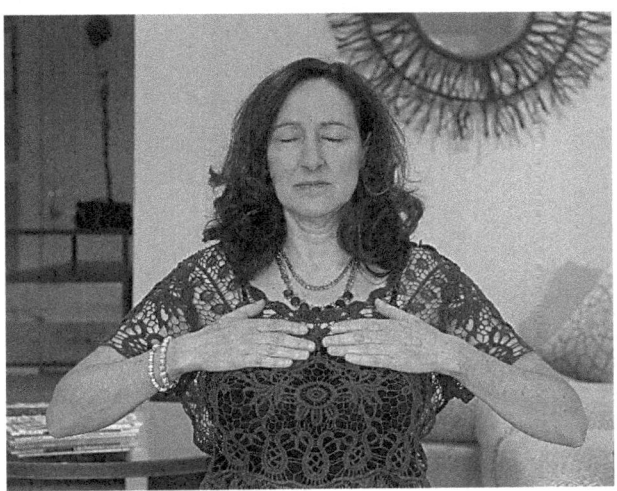

Chakra 4

Place your hands on your chest. Imagine your heart chakra is cleansing and clearing all that is no longer needed and allowing in the energy of a balanced, healthy heart chakra.

Chakra 5 is the throat chakra. It is located in the center of your throat; its color is sky blue. It is the center for speaking your truth, clarity of speaking, your voice, and expressing your true self. You are speaking your truth, your dogs are barking, your cats are meowing.

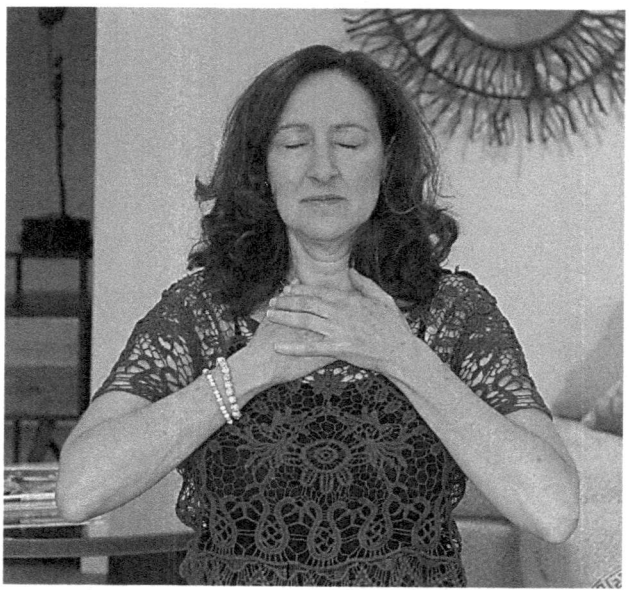

Chakra 5

Place your hands on your throat. Imagine your throat chakra is cleansing and clearing all that is no longer needed and allowing in the energy of a balanced, healthy throat chakra.

Chakra 6 is the third eye chakra. It is located in the center of your forehead; its color is indigo blue. This is your center of intuition, your clarity; 360-degree vision. As humans, a lot of the time we are "in our heads." You may have heard the saying, "Shift from your head to your heart," or "Get grounded." As this chakra opens, it brings the energies from all of the mental activity down into your heart center and your root chakra, opening your being to be connected with the present moment here on the Earth.

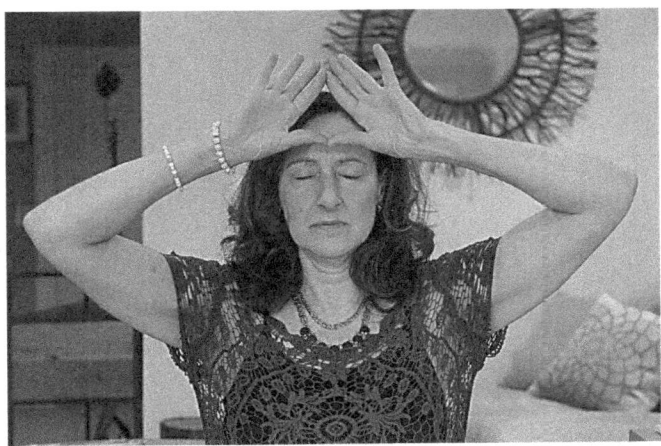

Chakra 6

Place your hands on your forehead. Imagine your third eye chakra is cleansing and clearing all that is no longer needed and allowing in the energy of a balanced, healthy third eye chakra.

Chakra 7 is the crown chakra. It is located on the top of your head; its color is light purple or white with gold. This is your connection center to God, Source, Higher Power, Universe, whatever that term is to you. When this chakra is open, you get crystal clear connection along with guidance and support.

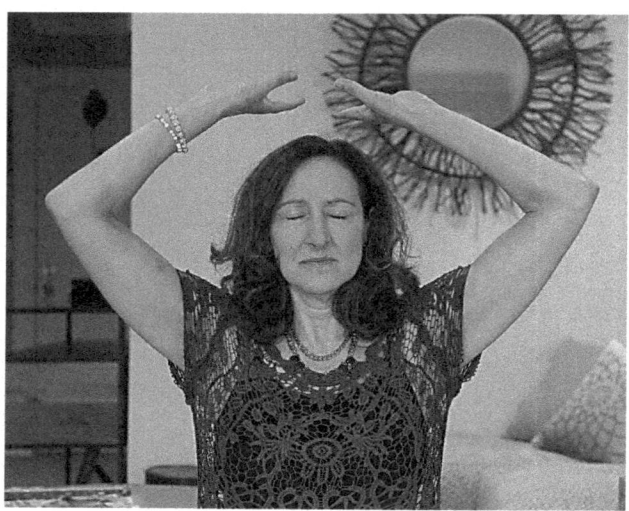

Chakra 7

Place your hands on the top of your head. Imagine your crown chakra is cleansing and clearing all that is no longer needed and allowing in the energy of a balanced, healthy crown chakra.

You now have your chakras a little more open and balanced than when we started. Doing this together with your animal helps you get in sync with one another, deepens connection, and enhances communication on multiple levels.

Check in and notice how you feel. Has there been a change in your body from when we started? Notice what those changes are.

You can open your eyes.

Now that you are grounded and balanced, the next thing to do is an assessment of your pet's chakras.

CHAPTER 14

Assessing the Chakras

NOW YOU ARE READY TO BEGIN the process of assessing, balancing, and checking your pet's chakras for a healing session.

The pendulum is a great tool to use while you are getting more and more in tune with your hands sensing the energy of the chakras. You will be guided to use the pendulum to read and assess each chakra before you do chakra balancing with your hands.

The pendulum is a tool with a visible outward expression to demonstrate the energy reading and state of the chakras, making it easy and clear for you to understand.

Here's what you will be doing for your pet's chakra healing session:

Chakra Healing Session Protocol

- Perform an assessment scan and document what the pendulum did on each chakra.

- Balance all seven of the chakras with the corresponding hand position. See Chapter 15, "Balancing the Chakras."

- Recheck chakras with the pendulum. Document the pendulum answers.

I have included both cat and dog chakra charts. Regardless of whether your pet is on his back or front, you have the chart to make your notes.

For your convenience, you can download 8 ½" x 11" charts with this QR code:

QR Code: Feline and Canine Chakra Charts

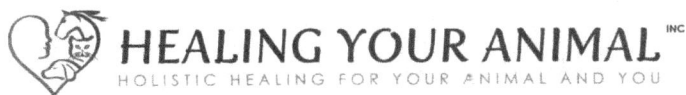

Feline Chakras

Chakra 6
Chakra 7

Chakra 5
Chakra 4

Chakra 3

Chakra 2
Chakra 1

Chakra 6
Chakra 7
Chakra 5
Chakra 4

Chakra 3

Chakra 2
Chakra 1

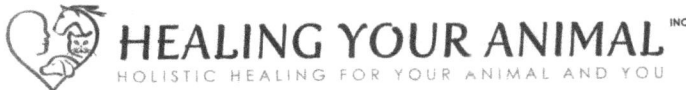

Canine Chakras

Chakra 6
Chakra 7
Chakra 5

Chakra 4

Chakra 3

Chakra 2
Chakra 1

Chakra 6
Chakra 7
Chakra 5

Chakra 4

Chakra 3

Chakra 2
Chakra 1

109

Assessing the Chakras

To learn how to use a pendulum, see the Appendix at the end of the book.

Before starting your chakra balancing session, you do an assessment with a pendulum to see the state of the seven main chakras before beginning.

Use your pendulum 2–4 inches above your pet's body over each of the seven chakras starting with the first chakra, the root chakra, and ending with the seventh chakra, the crown chakra.

Document your findings on the chart.

If you have never used a pendulum, or you want a refresher on using a pendulum, I have you covered. This section is for you.

Using the Pendulum to Check Chakras

Note: During your assessment of the chakras, if the pendulum is moving in a clockwise motion (in the northern hemisphere), it means your pet's chakra is open. The pendulum may swing in small, tight circles or large, swooping circles. You can tell how open the chakra is based on the width of the circle. (If you are in the southern hemisphere, the pendulum will be moving in a counterclockwise direction to indicate an open chakra.)

Place the pendulum over each chakra, starting from the root chakra at the base of the spine (near where the tail connects to your pet's body).

Ask the pendulum to show you the first chakra.

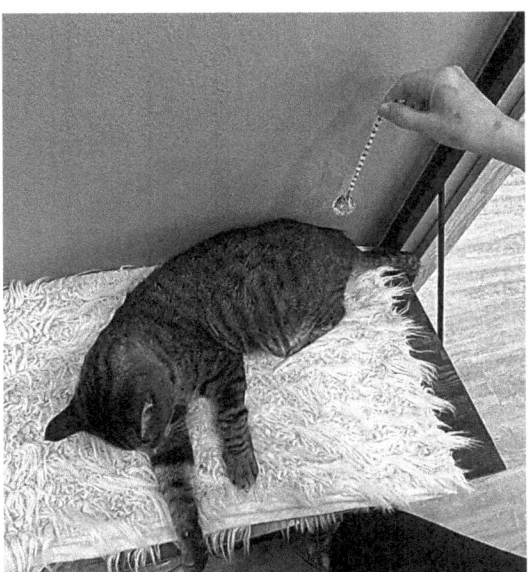

Pendulum Over The First Chakra

If the pendulum moves in the opposite direction of an open chakra, it means the chakra needs balancing.

If your pendulum is still and does not move, it means the chakra is blocked and needs opening.

If the pendulum moves in a diagonal or side to side motion, it means the chakra needs balancing.

Continue up the chakras to check them. Move your pendulum over each chakra, asking it to show you the corresponding number of the chakra you are checking, the same as you did for the first chakra.

Ask the pendulum to show you the second chakra.

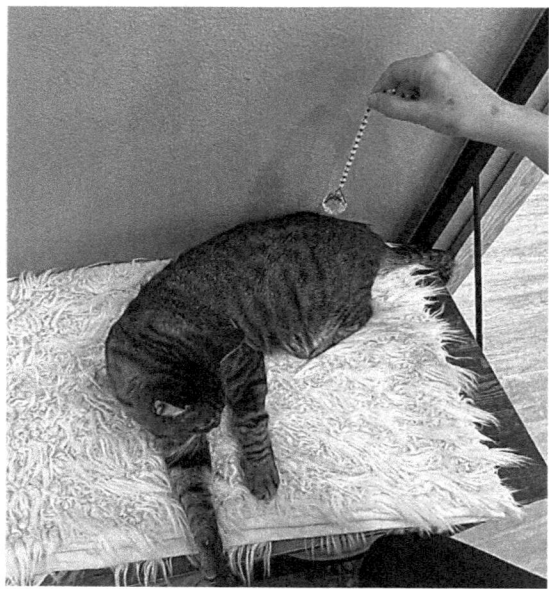

Pendulum Over the Second Chakra

Ask the pendulum to show you the third chakra.

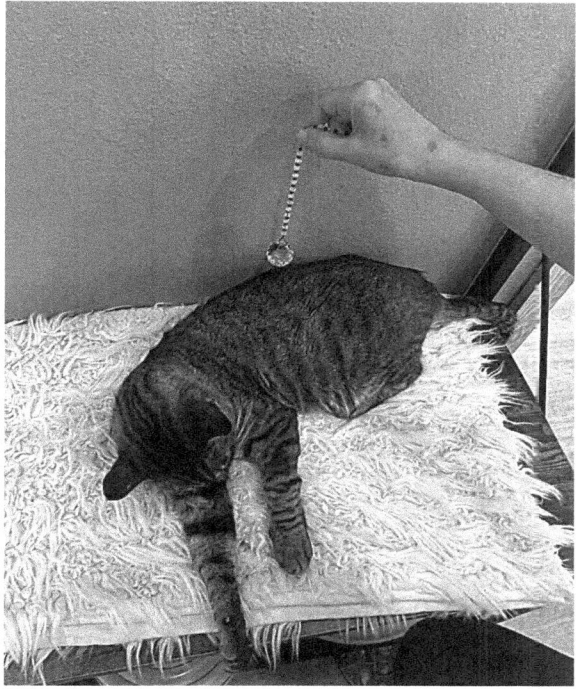

Pendulum Over the Third Chakra

Ask the pendulum to show you the fourth chakra.

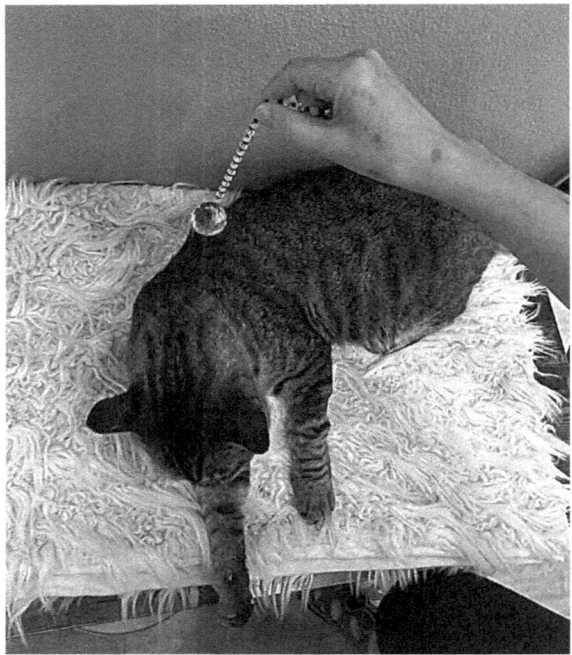

Pendulum Over the Fourth Chakra

Ask the pendulum to show you the fifth chakra.

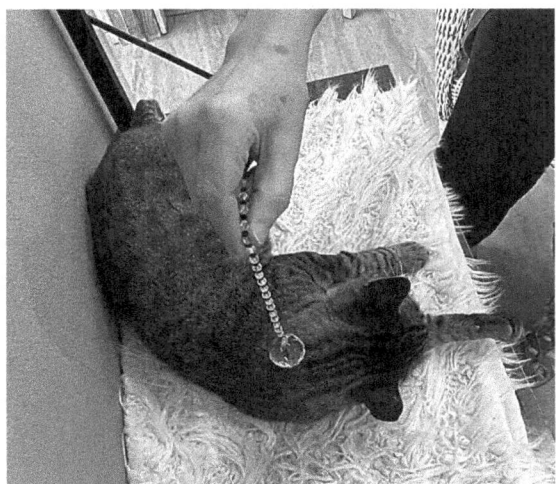

Pendulum Over the Fifth Chakra

Ask the pendulum to show you the sixth chakra.

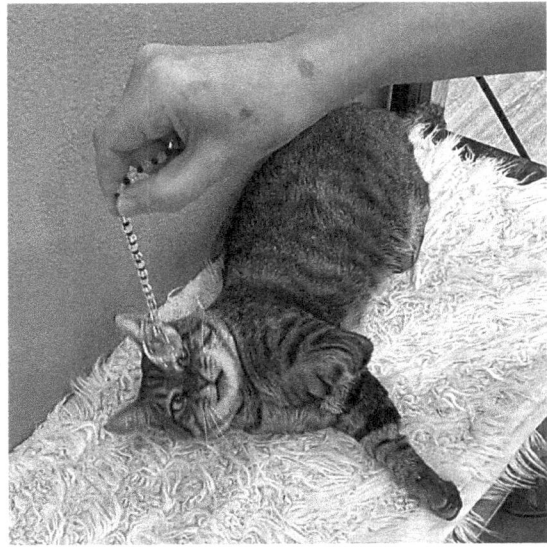

Pendulum Over the Sixth Chakra

Ask the pendulum to show you the seventh chakra.

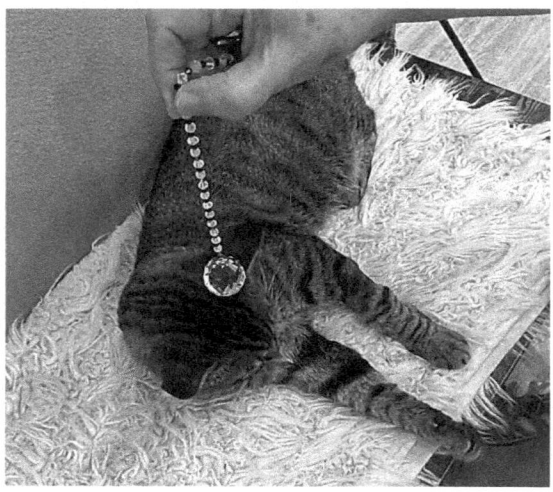

Pendulum Over the Seventh Chakra

Document your findings on the chart for each chakra.

Now that you have your assessment of your pet's chakras completed, it's time to balance your pet's chakras. Let's go!

CHAPTER 15

Balancing the Chakras

NOW THAT YOU KNOW WHICH CHAKRAS ARE IN BALANCE and which chakras are blocked or out of balance, it is time to balance your pet's chakras.

When doing a healing session with your pet, there are a few things to be aware of.

Ground Yourself

See the grounding exercise in Chapter 13, "Preparing You."

Use Two-Handed Connection

When working with your pet, always use two-handed connection. (When one hand is working a specific spot, it doesn't matter where the second hand rests as long as there is a connection with your pet's body.)

Two-handed connection is my preferred and recommended method to do with your pet(s).

- It reinforces connection and bonding time with the two of you.

- The hand positions provide powerful, effective chakra balancing.

- You feel and know when something is different with your pet.

Now you are ready to begin working with your pet. Something to keep in mind when working with your animal is that there may be times you don't stay fully grounded. Here is what to pay attention to. The signs you are not fully grounded are when you feel:

- Nauseous
- Shaky
- Feeling energy coming into your hand, arm, and/or body

What to do if this happens:

Pause, disconnect, ground yourself, and then reconnect with your animal.

Know the Signs of Release

Doing healing work with your pet, it is important to watch your pet's behavior because you may not always feel the shifts happening in your pet's body. Some ways your pet may show you that energy has moved:

- Wiggle
- Relaxed stretch

- Deep sigh
- Yawn
- A change in breathing pattern

Being consciously in the moment allows you to see these signs more easily.

Hand Position Method

Start with the first chakra (root chakra), at the base of the spine, where the tail connects to your pet's back.

Gently place your hands on the root chakra, with a pressure the weight of half pound or less.

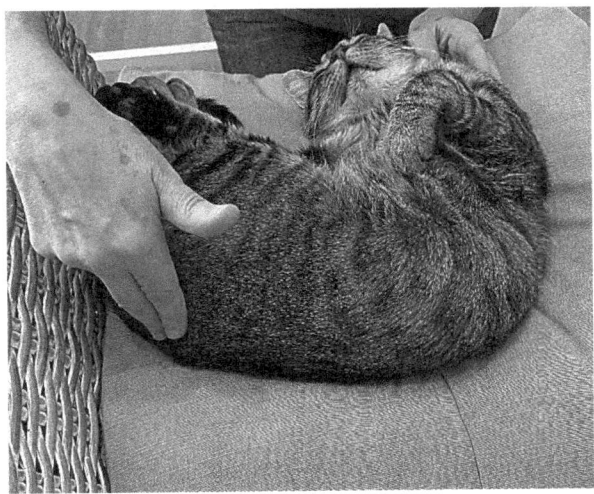

Hand Position for the First Chakra

Note: If you have a cat or small dog, you may want to use two fingers rather than your whole hand. If you are using your whole hand on your cat or small dog, you are accessing both the first and second chakras.

Notice what is happening under your hands. If the area is hot, that means there is more energy there than needed; the chakra is overactive. Something is causing the energy to pool in this chakra. If the area is cold, there is not enough energy, and the chakra is underactive. The area needs more energy to get it back into balance.

A balanced chakra has a nice open, flowing feeling. If you are really in tune, you may feel the clockwise/counterclockwise spin of the chakra.

Hold this position for 20–30 seconds, until you feel a shift, or your pet gives a sign of release, whichever comes first.

Continue using the hand positions up the rest of the chakras of your pet's body to the crown chakra at the top of the head.

Note: the chakras can be balanced on the front of the body as well as the back of the body except for the crown, which is at the center of the top of the head. Sometimes your pet will roll over and want the front of his/her body balanced. Notice this and honor them by balancing their front too.

Do this for the rest of the seven chakras.

Location of the second chakra:

- Back: midline over the hips on the low back

- Front: just below the belly button, between the waist and pelvis

As I previously explained, typically, cat and dog belly buttons appear as flat scars without hair, located in the middle of the abdomen, midway between the abdomen and the hips.

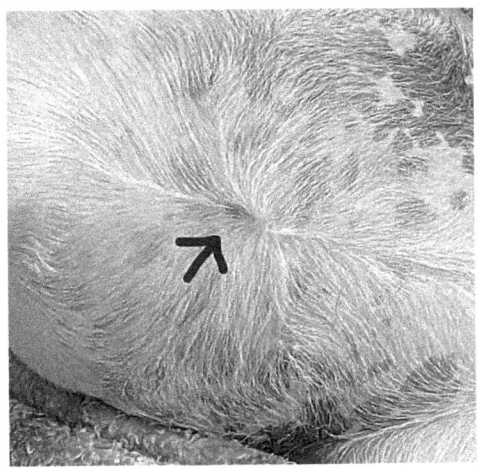

Gracie the Beagle's Belly Button

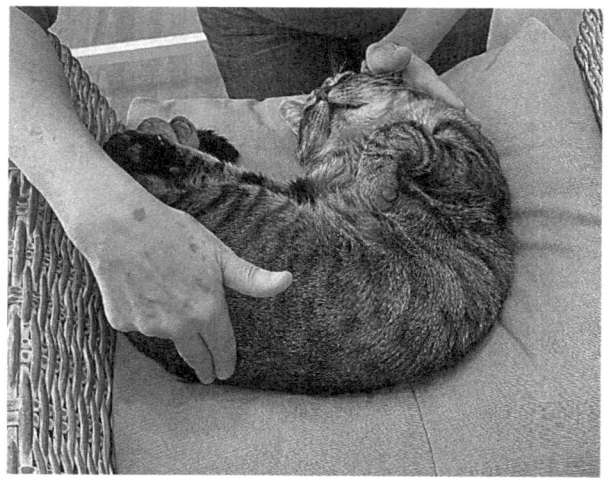

Hand Position for the Second Chakra

Location of the third chakra:

- Back: mid-back
- Front: between the base of the ribcage and above the navel

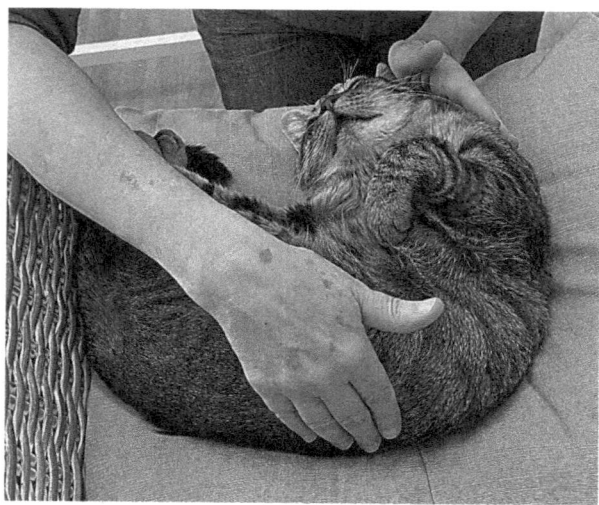

Hand Position for the Third Chakra

Location of the fourth chakra:

- Back: between the shoulders
- Front: center of chest

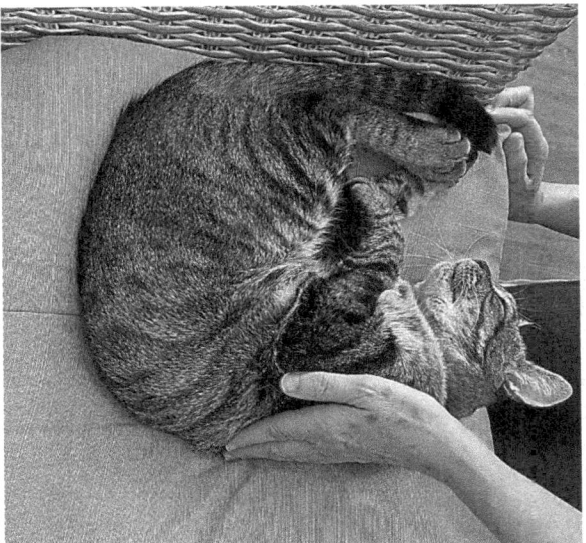

Hand Position for the Fourth Chakra, on the Back

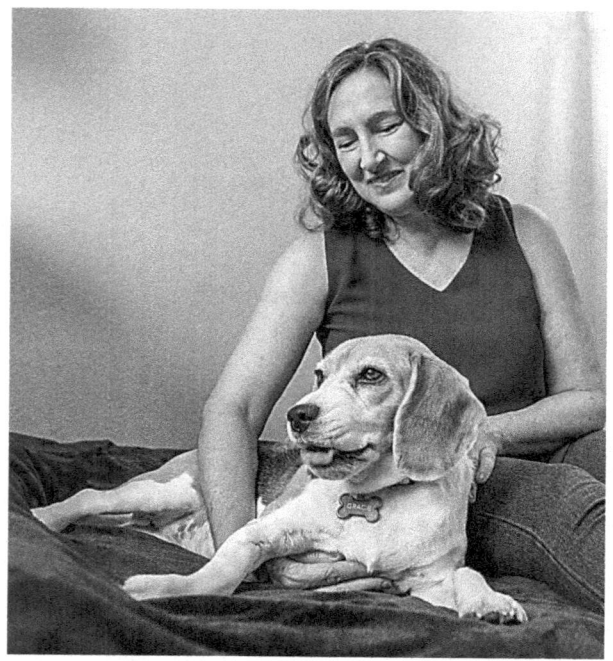

Hand Position for the Fourth Chakra, Front and Back Together

Location of the fifth chakra:

- Back: back of the neck
- Front: center of the neck

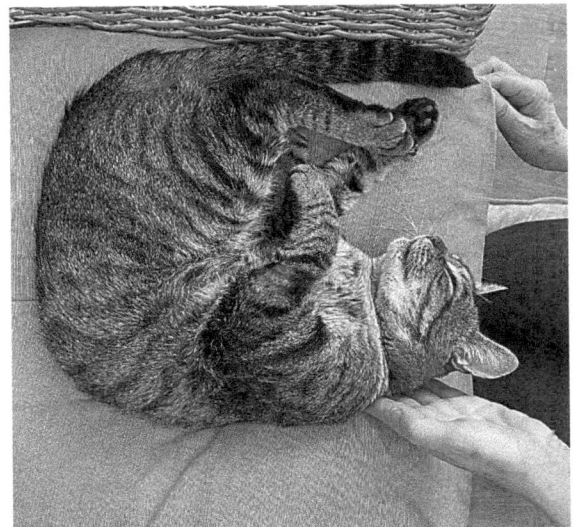

Hand Position for the Fifth Chakra

Location of the sixth chakra:

- Back: back of the head
- Front: center of the forehead

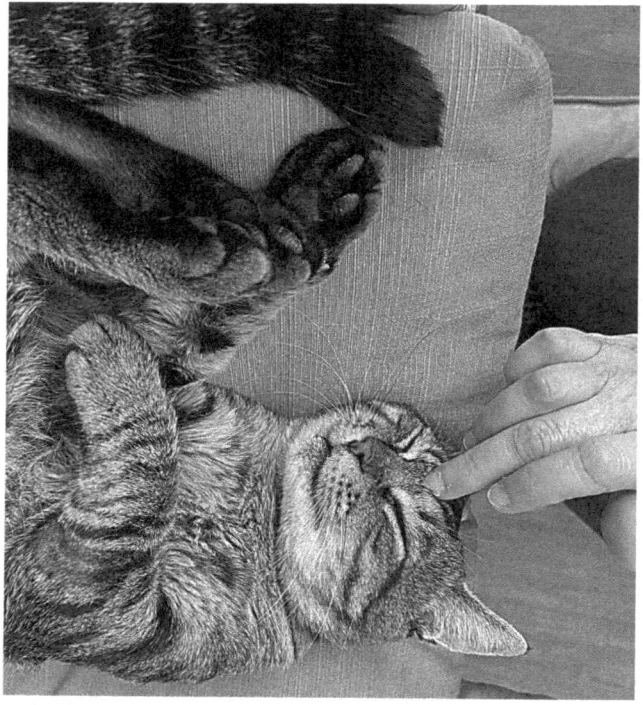

Hand Position for the Sixth Chakra

Location of the seventh chakra: top of the head in the center in front of the bump (external occipital protuberance).

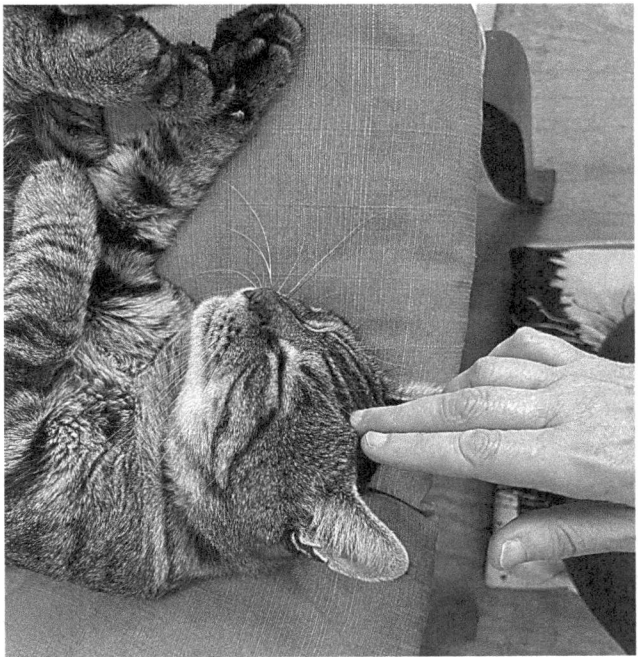

Hand Position for the Seventh Chakra

Once you have all seven chakras supported with the hand positions, then use your pendulum to check the chakras one through seven up the body as you did in Chapter 14, "Assessing the Chakras."

Document your observations on the chart. Notice what changed by doing the chakra balancing.

If there are chakras still blocked or out of balance, repeat the hand position on the respective chakras and check with your pendulum until you have all chakras open, balanced, and flowing optimally for your pet's well-being.

Enhanced Chakra Balancing

After you get used to balancing your pet's chakras, here are some ways to enhance your pet's chakra balancing with sound, color, crystals, and essences.

Adding Sound

You always have your hands and your voice with you. This can be an easy addition to your pet chakra balancing session.

While holding each of the seven hand positions on the respective seven chakras, chant the sound associated with each chakra. The vibration will give both of you a balancing.

Note: if you pet is shy and skittish, consider using a whisper, very low noise, or hum quietly in your head to have the same healing impacts or skip using sound vibration altogether.

Adding Color with Visualization

As you hold each hand position, visualize the respective vibrant chakra color with each chakra.

It is important to remember *vibrant* colors. The chakra colors are the vibrant rainbow colors in a healthy balanced state. In one of my recent Pet Chakra Classes, two of my students had big aha moments when they realized the importance of visualizing vibrant colors. They each had different responses to working with the vibrant colors.

For one, it helped her speed up as she was aligned matching the energy and frequencies of the colors.

For the other, it helped her slow down and wait for the chakra to shift from dull red to vibrant red, dull orange to vibrant orange, etc., through the chakra balancing with her pet.

Adding Color with Physical Items

If your pet has a chakra that is having trouble balancing and staying in balance, you can have your pet wear a bandana, a shirt, etc., of the respective chakra color to support the chakra balancing with color vibration.

You can put a towel or blanket of the respective chakra color down in your pet's bed or favorite place to support the chakra balancing with color vibration. Feel free to get creative.

Adding Healing Your Animal Essences

Essences definition: A substance considered to possess a high degree of the predominant qualities of a natural

129

product (as a plant or drug) from which it is extracted (as by distillation or infusion). "Healing Your Animal and Healing You" (formerly called Vi Miere) essences are created and handcrafted using the healing properties of crystals, minerals, flowers, and nature.

There is chakra essence set available to help balance your and your pet's chakras. The chakra essences are available to purchase individually or as a set. The set comes with an additional essence that seals in the balanced chakras and it comes with a guided meditation with sound healing through the seven main chakras for full chakra balancing.

HealingYourAnimal.com/MistsForPeople.php

Additional Chakras

The one thing I have found consistent studying the chakras is most people agree on the seven main chakras in the body that align with the colors and light vibrations of the rainbow. I have discussed my personal and professional experiences working with the seven main chakras in your body and your pet's body.

Depending on what source you refer to, there are a variety of ways of numbering and ordering additional chakras. It's not that any one of these is wrong, just that they are using a different system. At this point it is up to you to discern the different systems and how the information will help you because each system contains valuable information.

I am addressing a few of the additional chakras in this chapter to assist you in diving deeper into learning about chakras.

Bud Chakras

Bud chakras are the next most important chakras for your pet. Bud chakras consist of the four paws and the base of the ears as they open out from the head. They are especially receptive to subtle energy vibrations such as changes in the weather like a thunderstorm, or even impending, major earth events like an earthquake or hurricane.

Paw Chakras

Each of your pet's paws has a chakra.

When open, your pet is connected to the Earth and the energy grids of the Earth. They are in close connection and harmony with the Earth. Your pet is also able to discharge excess energy that isn't serving it into the Earth (grounding).

Your dog may kick dirt with its paws, a way of sending his/her scent into the world.

Your cat will dig to cover his/her waste, connecting with the Earth and hiding their scent.

To balance the paws, simply hold the pendulum over each paw beforehand, to see if it is in or out of balance or blocked. Then hold your hand over the top of your pet's paws one at a time to balance or unblock them. Check with the pendulum afterward to see if all four paws are now in balance. Continue holding your hand over each paw until all four paws are balanced. Confirm they are in balance with your pendulum.

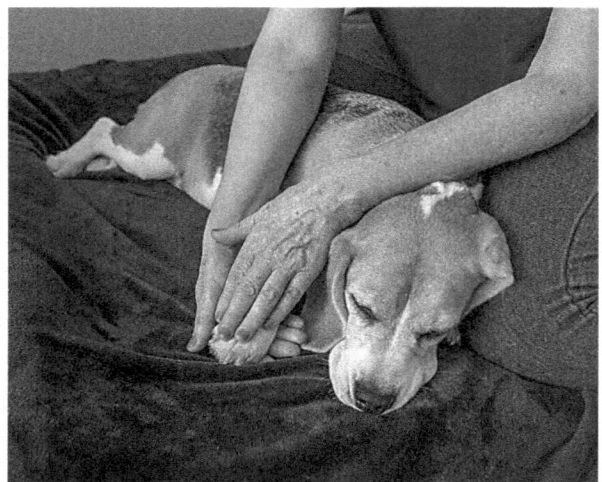

Gracie's Paw Chakra

Ear Chakras

The ear chakras are located at the base of ears. They help your cat or dog hear to their full range.

These chakras can become out of balance, closed, or blocked due to:

- High-pitched noises
- Stress
- Ear infections (side effect)

These imbalances can cause your pet to be agitated, anxious, or depressed.

Note: Cats can hear sounds an octave higher than dogs and 1.6 octaves higher than humans.

To balance the ears, simply hold the pendulum over each ear opening beforehand, to see if it is in or out of balance or blocked. Hold your hand lightly over the area in front of your pet's ear openings one at a time.

Note: if your pet is sensitive in this area, you may want to hold your hand two inches off the body, above the ear opening.

Hold for 20 seconds or until your pet shifts or shows a sign of release, whichever comes first. Check with the pendulum afterward to see if both ears are now in balance.

Ear Chakra Balancing Calming After Fourth of July Fireworks

Roxy, a Maltese dog, came in for a session at the veterinarian clinic after the Fourth of July fireworks. Her guardian, Lori, said that Roxy was so anxious. Nothing worked, not her thunder shirt, cannabis treats, or a prescription sedative. Roxy was shaking to her core and wouldn't settle. She had been on edge with noises setting off her anxiety ever since the fireworks occurred two weeks prior.

When I worked her ear chakras, she immediately responded, laid down, and settled into a deep calm. Roxy's guardian was relieved and commented that this was the calmest she had seen Roxy in a while. Her ear chakras had gotten overstimulated with the loud booms of fireworks and needed rebalancing. This balancing was a great relief to Roxy. Afterward, her eyes looked clearer, her face was softer, and her guardian commented that she had her Roxy back.

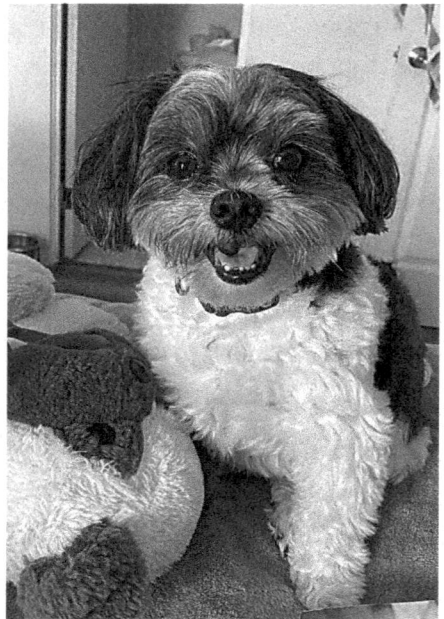

Roxy

CHAPTER 16

Healthy, Free, and Harmonious

NOW THAT YOU'VE BEEN ON THIS JOURNEY of discovering that your pet has chakras that affect their health, behavior, and quality of life and how to balance them, I encourage you to make this a regular part of your time with your precious pet.

I recommend making this a daily practice for you and a weekly practice for your pet to keep you and your pet living your best lives.

- Make a commitment to yourself for regular grounding and chakra balancing.

- Decide the best time for you to practice, in the morning, afternoon, or evening.

- Make a commitment to your pet for regular chakra balancing.

- Set a day and time each week on your calendar now to balance your pet's chakras and honor that time; this will make balancing your pet's chakras simple and routine.

This time with you doing chakra balancing is important to your pet. If you set the day and time on your calendar for time with your pet and you don't honor it, your pet will know. Your pet may act out to get your attention.

I had this happen to one of my students who was not going to keep her commitment for a healing session with her dog. Her dog started acting out in ways she had never seen before. She quickly honored their time agreement, so both were happy. She was amazed to discover how important it was to her dog.

This is quality time with your pet with healthy benefits.

The benefit of you getting into the habit of balancing your chakras daily sets the tone for your day and your pet's day. Your pet looks to you for guidance of feeling safe and balanced.

Once you make balancing your chakras a daily habit, it will be easier to get back into the rhythm if you wander away from it. It's easier to get back into a habit rather than create the habit in the first place. Be patient with yourself.

The more you do the chakra balancing, the quicker you will be. Also, you can do a quick tune-up, and when you have more time, you can do a longer session. The important part is doing it.

Let's celebrate! You now know how to balance your chakras and your pet's chakras!

More Techniques

The techniques in this book with chakra balancing are a key practice to help you and your pets live healthy, free, and harmonious.

For more techniques on how to help you and your precious pet live your best lives, full of health, harmony, and happiness, I invite you to check out my first two books:

Bridging True Love Connection & Healing Between You and Your Animals teaches you proven, powerful techniques so you can connect more deeply with your pets to live healthier, happier lives together.

This book is great for:

- Helping you understand your pet better.
- Helping calm anxious, unsettled, hyper pets.
- Helping multiple pets in a household get along better.
- And more...

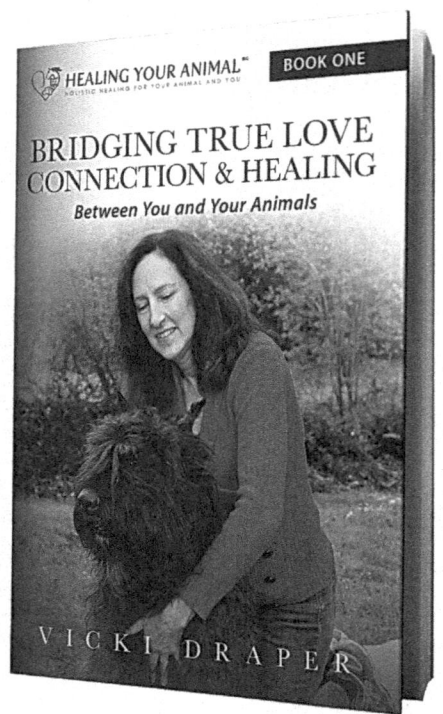

Vicki's First Book

Heart to Heart: How you can heal your animal through all stages of life empowers you as a pet guardian with tools for a deeper connection and better health.

It takes you on a journey through the life cycle of your pet. No matter what stage of life your pet is in, this book has something to offer you, even through the death process.

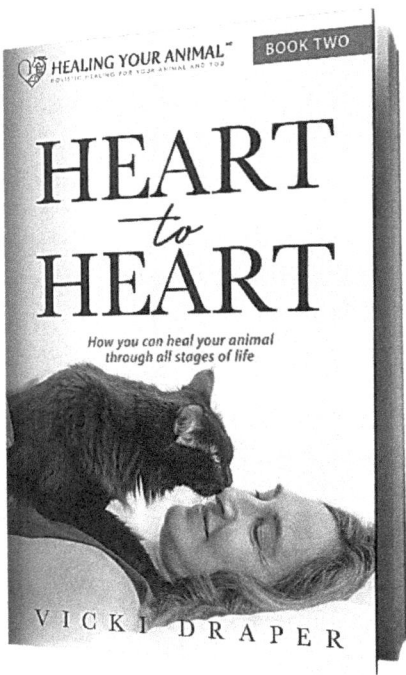

Vicki's Second Book

It doesn't matter if you are reading this book first. Each book in this series adds different healing techniques. Each book can be used on its own or you can add more techniques by reading all of them.

What's Next?

When I started writing this third book about the chakras, I did not know what my next book was going to be.

One day, I realized that the common thread through all my books, my teachings, and my healing practice is that healing starts with you, the pet guardian, the pet parent.

I am now writing a whole book dedicated to you, with techniques to help you shift from chaos to calm so you have better reactions to life experiences and a better quality of life and so you can be the best pet parent.

Anytime you are dealing with your pet and your pet's health, it starts with you. It's like on the airplane, they instruct you to put your oxygen mask on first before tending to your child or anyone else.

The same goes here with healing and being your pet's best parent. You take care of you. This also applies to taking care of your partner/spouse, child/children, family, and friends. It all starts with you.

I used to have a lot of anxiety, and I really didn't like being on edge all the time. When I learned grounding and chakra balancing (along with more techniques) it was a game changer for me.

I discovered that most of the anxiety I was feeling wasn't even mine. It turns out I was taking in the anxiety of the people around me and didn't realize it. And there were a lot of anxious people around.

I am so much calmer and happier as a result of regular grounding and chakra balancing.

I balance my chakras daily. I have found t makes a big difference in the quality of each day. It sets the tone for my day being in a calm, grounded, and present state. And if something throws me off, I can simply balance my chakras to recalibrate back into equilibrium. I have found balancing my chakras before bedtime also helps me have better quality of sleep.

It is a simple, powerful technique that has given me much freedom in my life.

On my trip home from taking Miranda, my daughter, back to college. I had left the hotel with a time buffer to get to the airport. I ended up in a traffic jam. The traffic on the interstate came to a full stop and was not moving.

Not knowing how long I'd be sitting there, I started to get all upset, thinking I might miss my flight. My thoughts were, "Why didn't I go with the known route instead of taking a different route? I should have, and then I wouldn't be stuck here. If only I'd left earlier, I wouldn't have gotten caught in this jam. I'm going to miss my flight! what if I miss my flight? I can't miss my flight!" Panic was setting in.

Before regular grounding and chakra balancing (and more healing techniques I have to share), I would have stayed in this stressful swirl of tension and beating myself up throughout my day. This time, I was able to catch myself quickly and stop, ground, and get clear on my options. I looked out at a beautiful sunrise happening as I was sitting there not moving on the interstate. I called the airline to see what my options were if I missed my flight. I also had the realization that if I had left a few minutes earlier, it could have been me in the wreck instead of just being stalled on the highway. I turned to gratitude. I would rather be sitting stalled in my vehicle than being in a car accident. I had the information I needed from the airlines. Now it was about calmly enjoying the moment, going with the flow of the situation. It wasn't long before traffic started moving slowly. It was down to one lane of cars on the shoulder, passing a five-car pileup. Once I was past that, the interstate was open, and traffic was flowing fully. I was able to easily make my flight. I appreciated being in a calm demeanor instead of feeling nervous and anxious.

My regular grounding and chakra balancing practice helped me get out of fight-or-flight quickly, get grounded, and have a much more pleasant experience.

Spirit and Sapphire, my cats, are more settled, happier, and harmonious as a result.

This is why I recommend you doing the grounding and chakra balance practice daily.

Writing a book dedicated to you helps your pet so that you both are living with health, harmony, and happiness during your time together.

This is my mission and calling, to help you and your pet live your best lives together.

If you are ready to have more calm in your life, I invite you to look for my next book: *Pet Parent's Guide to Self-*

Care: How you can have more ease and harmony in your life.

It has truly been an honor to join you in support of having you and your pet be healthy, free and harmonious.

—Vicki Draper, Author, Certified Healer, and Animal Communicator

Sending you many hugs with lots of love, purrs, and woofs!

Appendix

How to Use a Pendulum

Definition

A pendulum is a weight suspended from string or chain so that it can swing freely.

Also, an ancient tool for dowsing.

Why Use a Pendulum?

When working with a pendulum, you are asking questions of your higher self, the part of you connected to the infinite intelligence and wisdom of the cosmos.

When starting to build your scanning skill, it can be helpful to use a pendulum to see the physical representation of energy. You can easily see where the energy is flowing, blocked, sluggish, or unbalanced.

Pendulum Use Exceptions

- If you are in a hurry or determined that you already know what the pendulum will do, you will be affecting the results and you won't have a clear reading. This is not the time to be working with your pendulum.

- If you in a bad mood, it is not the time to be working with your pet or the pendulum.

- The pendulum never replaces the need for medical advice and veterinary care. If you pet has a health concern, please take them to the veterinarian.

Selecting Your Pendulum

You can create a pendulum from a string and washer from your toolbox. In 1993 Deepak Chopra demonstrated a pendulum made out of string and a washer on Oprah Winfrey's national television show.

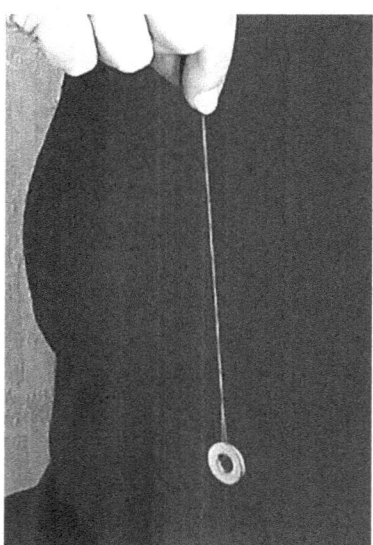

Pendulum made with washer and thread

You can make or buy beautiful pendulums made of beads and crystals.

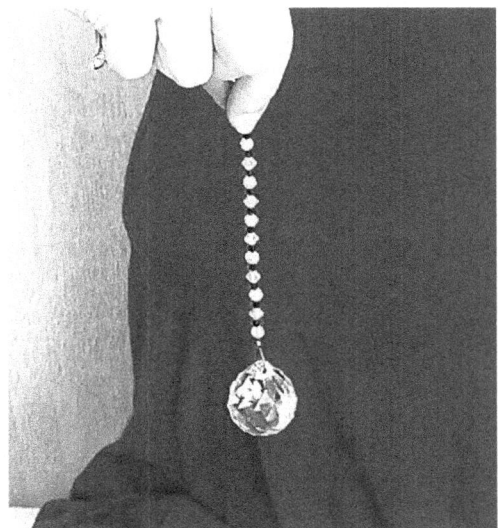

Pendulum made with crystal and beads

You can even use a necklace on a chain with a pendant.

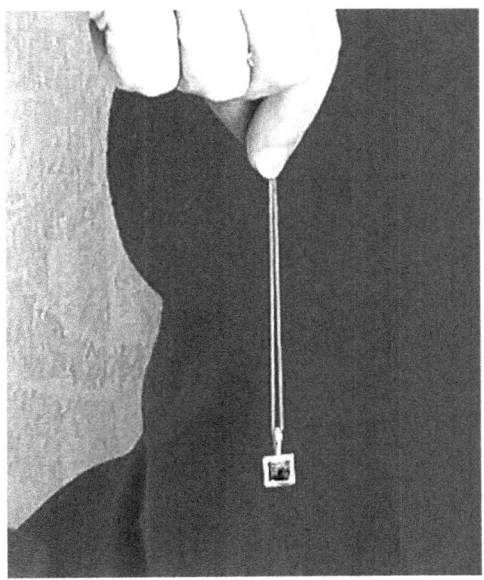

Pendulum Made With Necklace on Chain

Connecting with Your Pendulum

Make sure you are connected with your pendulum before you begin using it.

To connect with your pendulum:

- Ground yourself before starting to work with your pendulum. (See the grounding exercise in chapter 13.)

- Clear your head and be in an open mind. Taking a few deep centering breaths will help.

- Hold the string/chain in your dominant hand between thumb and index finger with the pendulum hanging down.

- Hold your elbow up to the side, above your heart and your hand for better flow of energy.

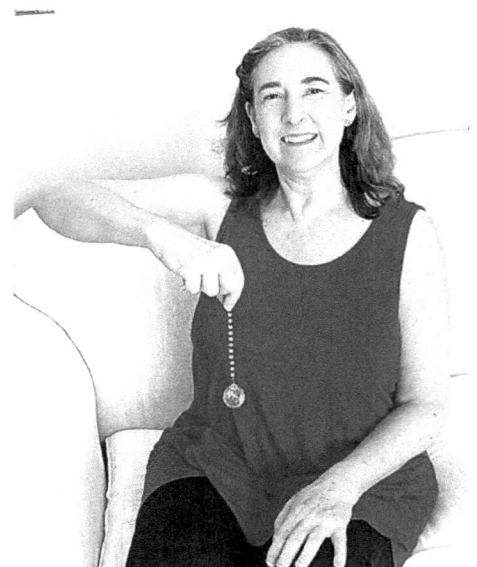

Pendulum Position for Optimal Energy Flow

- Ask it to show you a "yes" to see what happens.

- Ask it to show you a "no" to see what happens.

- Ask it to show you what "need more information" looks like.

- Test the pendulum with a "yes" question. Ask a question you know the name of such as "Is my name <your name>?"

- It will show you the same activity as it did when showing you a yes above. If it does not, then you need to start over, calibrating your pendulum to a consistent yes.

Once the pendulum is aligned and answering properly:

- Test the pendulum with a "no" question. Example: "Is my name <a random name>?" It will show you the same activity as it did when showing you a no above. If it does not, then you need to start over, calibrating your pendulum to a consistent no.

Now you are ready to ask your pendulum questions about the chakras.

Introducing the Pendulum to Your Pet

Before doing your assessment, it is important to introduce the pendulum to your pet. Hold it up and let them sniff it and see it. Then slowly move it to start assessing the chakras.

149

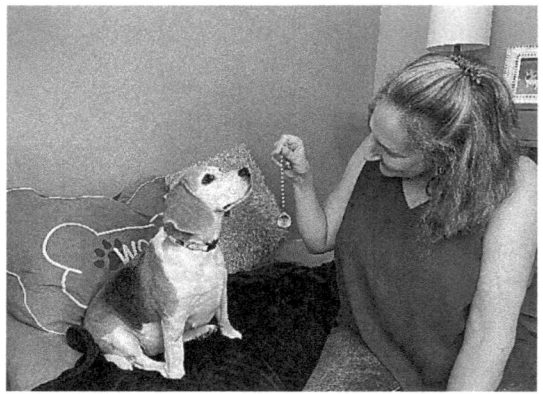

Vicki Introducing a Pendulum to Gracie

Be mindful when introducing the pendulum to your kitten or cat that they will be curious and bat at it with their paws. This is natural. Once you are past the curious stage, your kitten or cat will warm up to the pendulum and let you assess their chakras.

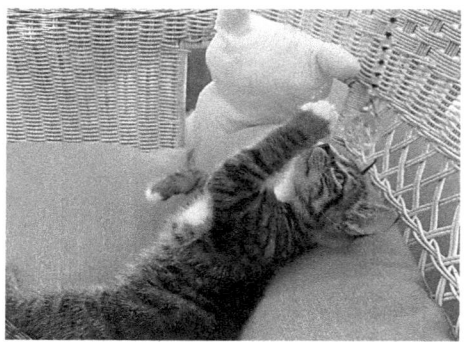

Vicki Introducing a Pendulum to Kitten El Tigre

Resources

"Governing Vessel – Points, Definition, and Case Study for Increasing Energy"
https://taichibasics.com/how-the-governing-vessel-can-increase-your-energy-points-definition-and-case-study/

"Large-Scale Effectiveness Trial of Reiki for Physical and Psychological Health"
https://pubmed.ncbi.nlm.nih.gov/31638407/

"What Are False Pregnancies in Dogs?"
https://pets.webmd.com/dogs/what-is-false-pregnancy-in-dog

"Why do cats get crystals in their urine?"
https://firstvet.com/us/articles/why-do-cats-get-crystals-in-their-urine

About the Author

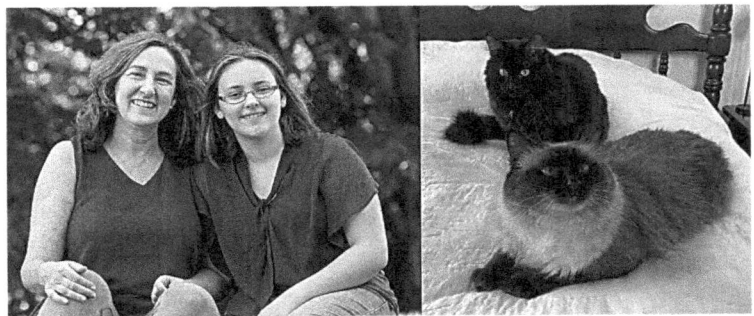

Vicki Draper with Daughter Miranda, and Cats Spirit and Sapphire

Vicki Draper is a highly regarded modern-day animal healer and author who supports family animals with health, harmony, and ease addressing wellness during every stage of your animal's life. With her skill set, she serves people locally and remotely, nationally, and internationally.

She is featured in multiple books and magazines and is the creator of healing products sold around the country and around the world. A natural-born animal communicator, Vicki's qualifications as a healer for both people and animals include being a licensed massage practitioner, a certified acupressurist and Reiki Master/Teacher, and training in craniosacral therapy.

Vicki deepened her connection with spirituality and was called to become a Science of Mind Prayer Practitioner with the Center for Spiritual Living in Seattle. She is trained and licensed to support others to face life challenges through affirmative prayer, which helps her better serve animals and their human families.

Vicki lives in the Greater Seattle Area with her two cats, Spirit and Sapphire, and Miranda when she is visiting from college. She loves to walk in nature daily, connecting with herons, eagles, and wildlife, bringing nature's wisdom into her life and healing practice.

If you would like further assistance with yourself or your animals, Vicki invites you to schedule a Healing Your Animal Assessment, to discuss your issues and concerns and together determine the best plan of support.

Connect with Vicki at HealingYourAnimal.com

Made in USA North Chelmsford, MA
1359525_9780997635027
02.10.2023 0729